Advances in Anatomy
Embryology and Cell Biology

Vol. 128

George Székely Clara Matesz

The Efferent System of Cranial Nerve Nuclei: A Comparative Neuromorphological Study

With 18 Figures

Springer-Verlag
Berlin Heidelberg New York
London Paris Tokyo
Hong Kong Barcelona
Budapest

Prof. Dr. George Székely
Dr. Clara Matesz

Department of Anatomy, University Medical School
4012 Debrecen, Hungary

ISBN 3-540-56207-9 Springer-Verlag Berlin Heidelberg New York
ISBN 0-387-56207-9 Springer-Verlag New York Berlin Heidelberg

Library of Congress Cataloging-in-Publication Data
Székely, George.
The efferent system of cranial nerve nuclei: a comparative neuromorphological study / George Székely, Clara Matesz. p. cm. – (Advances in anatomy, embryology and cell biology; vol. 128) Includes bibliographical references and index.
ISBN 3-540-56207-9 (acid-free paper: Berlin)
ISBN 0-387-56207-9 (acid-free paper: New York)
1. Nerves, Cranial. 2. Efferent pathways. 3. Comparative neurobiology. I. Matesz, Clara. II. Title. III. Series: Advances in anatomy, embryology and cell biology; v. 128.
QL801.E67 vol. 128 [QM471] 574.4 s-dc20 [591.4′8] 92-35109

Typesetting: Best-set Typesetter Ltd., Hong Kong
Printing and binding: Konrad Triltsch, Würzburg

21/3130-5 4 3 2 1 0 – Printed on acid-free paper

Contents

Abbreviations

Add	adductor
CER	cerebellum
Cc	central canal
Cct	cricothyroideus
CI	colliculus inferior
CS	colliculus superior
C2	second cervical root of spinal cord
D	dorsal
dmX	dorsal motor nucleus of vagus nerve
eso	esophagus
EW	nucleus of Edinger-Westphal
HRP	horseradish peroxidase
IO	inferior oblique muscle of eyeball
IR	inferior rectus muscle of eyeball
l, L	lateral
Lar	laryngeal muscles
LR	lateral rectus muscle of eyeball
m	medial
mlf	medial longitudinal fasciculus
MR	medial rectus muscle of eyeball
n, nn	nucleus, nuclei
nspV	spinal nucleus of trigeminal nerve
nIII	motor nucleus of oculomotor nerve
nIV	motor nucleus of trochlear nerve
nV	primary motor nucleus of trigeminal nerve
nVa	accessory nucleus of trigeminal nerve
nVm	main nucleus of trigeminal nerve
nVI	main nucleus of abducens nerve
nVIa	accessory nucleus of abducens nerve
nVII	primary motor nucleus of facial nerve
nVIIa	accessory nucleus of facial nerve
nVIIm	main nucleus of facial nerve
nIX	motor nucleus of glossopharyngeal nerve
nX	motor nucleus of vagus nerve
nXI	nucleus of accessory nerve
nXII	nucleus of hypoglossal nerve

Ph	constrictor pharyngis
Pro	protractor
R	rostral
Retr	retractor
SAL	superior salivatory nucleus
SO	superior oblique muscle of eyeball
SOL	solitary tract and nucleus
SR	superior rectus muscle of eyeball
stap	stapedius neurons
sty	stylopharyngeus
sy	sympathetic neurons
TO	tectum opticum
tt	tensor tympani
tspV	spinal tract of trigeminal nerve
4th	fourth ventricle
V	trigeminal nerve
Vint	intermediate trigeminal subnucleus
Vv	ventral subnucleus of trigeminal nerve
VII	facial nerve
VIIv	ventral facial subnucleus
VIId	dorsal facial subnucleus
VIII	statoacoustic nerve
IX	glossopharyngeal nerve
X	vagal nerve
XI	accessory nerve
XII	hypoglossal nerve

1 Introduction

Since their description by Sömmering in 1778, the cranial nerves have been grouped into twelve pairs, to which a 13th pair, the nervus terminalis, was added 100 years later by Fritsch in 1878 (cited in Haller von Hallerstein 1934). The central pathway character of the first and second pair was soon recognized and that of the 13th pair is still a subject of debate with respect to whether it is an independent cranial nerve or part of the olfactoretinal system (Szabo 1991). In the present endeavor we confine the discussion to the efferent nuclei of the "real" cranial nerves which emerge from the brain stem. As the classification of these nerves and nuclei is strongly associated with the various "head theories," we start with a brief survey of them.

1.1 Theories Regarding the Evolution of the Head

As first formulated by Goethe, in 1790, in his famous *Kopftheorie* (see Goethe 1824) and later by Oken (1807), the skull is built up from equivalent structural elements derived from the vertebrae, and these elements are placed serially one after another. Although this *Wirbeltheorie* did not survive in its original form, it became the basis for a variety of segmental theories of head development proposed by comparative anatomists. Fundamental to these theories was the assumption that the mesoderm in the head region was segmented in a manner resembling that of the trunk region (Balfour 1878; Fürbringer 1897). Gegenbaur (1888) even compared the skeletal bars of visceral arches of the pharyngeal gut to the ribs of the trunk. Two types of segmentation were distinguished in the head region, the somitomeric and branchiomeric, with some disagreement about their relation to one another. The somitomers were homologized with the somites of the trunk region, and the lateral plate mesoderm was thought to continue in the branchiomers into which the body cavity extended forming the head cavities (Goodrich 1930).

While the synthesis of the posterior part of the head from the occipital segments was conclusively established, there were a few early opponents to the general segmental theory of the head, especially concerning the preotic region (Huxley 1858–59; Froriep 1902). The problem remained unsettled until Meier (1979, 1982) and associates (see Jacobson 1988) were able to show traces of segmentation of the preotic mesoderm with the aid of the scanning electron microscope in a variety of animal embryos. While these findings rehearsed the old thesis of head segmentation, the suggestion that the preotic somitomers, seven in some animals and four in others, were vestigial counterparts of trunk segments did not achieve general acceptance. The controversy was partly based on the failure to show preotic segmentation in amphibian (Youn and Malacinski 1981) and in fish (Kimmel et al. 1988) embryos and to match mesodermal segments with neuronal segments in the anterior head region (Sakai 1987). From a large body of comparative anatomical data, Gans and Northcutt (1983) came to the conclusion that the anterior portion of the skull was basically a de novo structure in verebrate evolution and that it was not serially homologous to any trunk structures. It is well known that a significant contingent of the head mesoderm is of neural crest origin (Le Douarin 1982), and it may be noteworthy in the present context that the expression of homeobox genes, which are responsible for the segmentation of the postotic region, has not yet been reported in cranial mesoderm derivatives (Holland 1988). Due to these controversies, head segmentation is still an open question.

1.2 The Classification of Cranial Nerves

The many kinds of classification found in the old and recent literature (Haller von Hallerstein 1934; Ariëns Kappers et al. 1936; Starck 1978) are of historical interest and accurately reflect the actual state of debate about the different head theories. We select the current scheme of classification which can be directly traced back to the segmental theory of the head.

This theory, as best known from the recent literature, is based on Goodrich's (1930) well-known "model" fish. This "animal" possesses three preotic, two vestigial metotic, and four postotic somitomeres. In analogy with the structure of the trunk, the segmented mesoderm gives rise to the "somatic" muscles in the head region, and the corresponding nerves are called somatomotor nerves and their nuclei somatomotor nuclei. The mesoderm of the branchial arches is the direct continuation of the lateral plate mesoderm of the trunk in this scheme. It is known that visceral muscles derive from the visceral leaf of the lateral plate mesoderm, consequently muscles originating from the branchial mesoderm are visceral muscles. They are, however, striated muscles, and in order to distinguish them from smooth visceral muscles of the trunk region, they receive the epithet "specific." Their nerves are specific visceromotor nerves, and the nuclei are called specific visceromotor nuclei.

In another classification scheme, the motor nuclei are termed according to their positions in the brain stem. The somatomotor nuclei are often called the dorsomedial nuclear column, whereas the specific visceromotor nuclei form the ventrolateral nuclear column. In the spinal cord, a group of efferent nerve cells, the sympathetic preganglionic neurons, is found dorsal to the spinal (somato-)motor column. In the brain stem, the parasympathetic preganglionic neurons are placed dorsal to the brain stem-specific visceromotor column, and in order to distinguish them from the specific visceromotor neurons they are called general visceromotor neurons. In neuroanatomy textbooks, they are grouped in well defined nuclei.

This type of classification has been transferred to the sensory side as well. Sensory nerves and their nuclei supplying the integumentum are designated as the general somatosensory system, whereas the 8th nerve, which conveys impulses from a sensory organ complex of ectodermal origin, is a specific somatosensory nerve. The entodermal mucous membrane of viscera is supplied by general viscerosensory nerves and usually they terminate in the viscerosensory nuclei.

There is a special visceral sensation, taste, which is not represented in the spinal cord. The taste buds (of ectodermal origin) are innervated by specific viscerosensory nerves which convey the impulse to specific viscerosensory nuclei.

1.3 Inconsistencies and Contradictions in the Classification of Cranial Nerves

First, a contradiction is apparent in the distinction of somatomotor and specific visceromotor muscles. The "somatomotor" tongue muscles of occipital myotome origin move a viscus, and the external eye muscles of undecided origin belong to the same category. Many of the muscles of branchial arch origin have no relation to viscera. It may be argued for the visceral character of the masticatory muscles, as they move a visceral skeleton, but the function and innervation of this muscle group is so exceedingly complex in animals with the secondary mandibular joint that it is difficult to compare to any visceral function in the conventional sense. It would be difficult to argue for the visceral character of the muscles of facial expression, the auditory muscles, and the muscles of the accessory nerve. Moreover, it has been shown that muscles associated with branchial arch skeletal structures are derived from paraxial mesoderm (Noden 1983).

A second logical fault relates to the first, that is, the location of vegetative nerve cells. In the spinal cord they are dorsal to the (somato-)motor column. In the brain stem there are two visceromotor columns, a specific and a general, and both are ventral to the somatomotor column. Obviously, it would be an oversimplification to insist on unfounded homologies and analogies in the structure of the spinal cord and brain stem.

Third, on the sensory side, the eighth nerve is a specific somatosensory nerve because it innervates a sense organ derived from the ectoderm. Nerves which innervate the taste buds are specific viscerosensory nerves, although the taste buds are also of ectodermal origin. One may argue that the taste buds are the receptors of a viscus therefore they are visceral sense organs; but the same line of argument is obviously denied of the tongue muscles.

Fourth, in the trigeminal nerve, the efferent side is represented by the specific visceromotor nucleus whereas the afferent side provides the general somatosensory supply to the skin of the face, the forehead and to the specific visceromotor muscles. Trigeminal branches contribute also to the general viscerosensory innervation of the tongue and oral cavity. Thus, somatic and visceral sensations converge upon the trigeminal sensory nuclei.

More scrutinous investigations would reveal more of such discrepancies in the classification of cranial nerves. Most of them could be avoided by changing the semantics. The primary aim of our effort is to propose a different classification by the incorporation of new data and the demonstration of new aspects in the evolution of cranial nerves. In this attempt, we rely mainly on our own data obtained from cobalt labeling studies of frogs, lizards, and rats, but they are richly supplemented by the observations of other authors made on different animal species. We focus on the efferent side of cranial nerves and in our classification we describe the morphological characteristics of neurons, their innervated periphery, and function.

2 Materials and Methods

The experiments were performed on the common frog, *Rana esculenta*, sand lizard, *Lacerta agilis*, and Wistar rats of both sexes. (The lizards were collected with permission of the Local Environmental Protection Agency, No. 91/1984.) Cranial nerves, except the first, second, and eighth or one of their peripheral branches, were labeled with a cobalt solution, either separately or in combination with other cranial nerves. In order to achieve the shortest route for cobalt transport the appropriate nerve was prepared at its closest point of emergence. Frogs and lizards were anesthetized with MS 222 (tricaine methane-sulfonate, Sigma) crystals applied to the frogs' skin and to the mucous membrane of the lizards' mouth. Rats were anesthetized by intraperitoneal administration of a 10% urethane solution (13 ml/weight kg).

In frogs, the nerves were usually exposed by an oropharyngeal incision at the mucous membrane of the roof of the mouth. The cranial cavity was opened by removal of a small portion of the base of the skull. The branches of the oculomotor and abducens nerves were exposed after removing the eyeball. The nerves of the jaw-opening and -closing muscles were prepared at the appropriate muscle according to the terminology of Gaupp (1896).

In lizards cranial nerves III and IV and the ophthalmic branch of the trigeminal nerve were exposed within the orbit after removing the eyeball. The abducens nerve was dissected through a pharyngeal approach by removing part of the hard palate and the base of the skull. The maxillary and mandibular divisions of the trigeminal nerve were prepared by removing the posterior jaw adductor, the pterygoid muscles, and the posterior part of the orbit. The facial nerve was found through the tympanic cavity and filled proximal to the geniculate ganglion. The glossopharyngeal, the vagoaccessory and the hypoglossal nerves were exposed in the postotic region by removing fragments of the surrounding bones.

In rats the cranial nerves III, IV, and VI and the ophthalmic division of the trigeminal nerve were found within the cavernous sinus after removing the cerebral hemisphere and the covering bones. The whole trigeminal nerve and its maxillary and mandibular divisions were filled within the cranial cavity after removing the masticatory muscles and the underlying bones. The facial nerve was followed to the brain stem by clipping away the bony facial canal. Cranial nerves IX–XII were found outside the cranial cavity (Green 1959) or, in a few cases, the nerves were dissected at their exit from the brain stem by removing a part of the occipital bone.

The proximal end of the dissected nerve was introduced into a fine glass or plastic tube containing the labeling solution. In frogs, either $CoCl_2$ or Co^{3+}Lys (a complex compound of Co^{3+} and l-lysine) was used in 0.11 *M* concentration (Görcs et al. 1979; Székely and Gallyas 1975; Urban and Székely 1983). In lizards and rats, the 0.11 *M* and 0.22 *M* Co^{3+}Lys solutions, respectively, were used. The tube was covered with a mixture of silicon oil and grease and fixed to the surrounding tissues with histoacryl blue. After a survival time of 1–3 days, the brain stem and the cervical part of the spinal cord was dissected and immersed for 10 min in a 0.11 *M* phosphate buffer solution saturated with H_2S. The specimens were fixed in 70% ethanol and embedded in paraffin. The 40 μm serial cross-sections were intensified with a physical developer (Görcs et al. 1979) and counterstained with nuclear fast red or toluidine blue. Serial sections of two normal brains from each species were stained with toluidine blue as controls. Reconstructions of the nuclei and neurons were made with the aid of a camera lucida attached to a Reichert microscope.

3 The Hypoglossal Nucleus: The Appearance of the Muscular Tongue

Since the acquisition of a muscular tongue is a relatively late event in evolution, there has been some confusion in the classification of the hypoglossal nerve. In tongueless fishes, a structure homologous to the hypoglossal nerve cannot be found, and this may be the reason that even recent comparative anatomy books (e.g., Starck 1982) do not list this nerve among cranial nerves. A definitive tongue with intrinsic muscles first appears in tetrapods and this coincides with the caudal enlargement of the cranium by the assimilation of the rostralmost vertebrae. Tongue muscles derive from the segmented occipital mesoderm, and their nerves are called the spino-occipital nerves in the early literature (Fürbringer 1897) suggesting their spinal cord origin. In neckless tetrapods, as most amphibia are, a number of other muscles differentiate from the same and subjacent segments and their innervation merges with that of the tongue. These nerves form the first spinal nerve and this is the basis of the old view about the spinal origin of the hypoglossal nerve. It becomes distinct first in mammals, but, as presented below, the hypoglossal nerve and its nucleus can be shown also in submammalian vertebrates possessing a muscular tongue.

3.1 Frog

If the first spinal nerve is soaked with cobalt, then labeling reveals a dorsomedial cell group in the obex region, motoneurons in the ventral horn of the first spinal cord segment, neurons in an intermediate position between these two groups, and small, presumably preganglionic, sympathetic neurons (Fig. 1a). This collection of neurons corresponds to the peripheral innervation of the first spinal nerve which in addition to tongue muscles supplies deep trunk muscles and the second ganglion sympathicum. If cobalt treatment is limited to the lingual branch of the first spinal nerve, then labeling is found only in the dorsomedial and in the intermediate motoneuron groups which correspond to the dorsomedial and lateral hypoglossal nuclei, respectively. The dorsomedial nucleus can be regarded as the nucleus proper of the hypoglossal nerve supplying the intrinsic tongue muscles and the genioglossus muscle, whereas the lateral nucleus innervates extrinsic tongue muscles (Stuesse et al. 1983).

The dorsomedial nucleus begins in the upper obex region and extends into the closed part of the medulla (Fig. 18a). The constituent neurons have oval- or spindled-shaped perikarya with a longitudinal diameter of 30–35 μm. A dorsal and a ventrolateral dendrite group originates from the pointed ends of

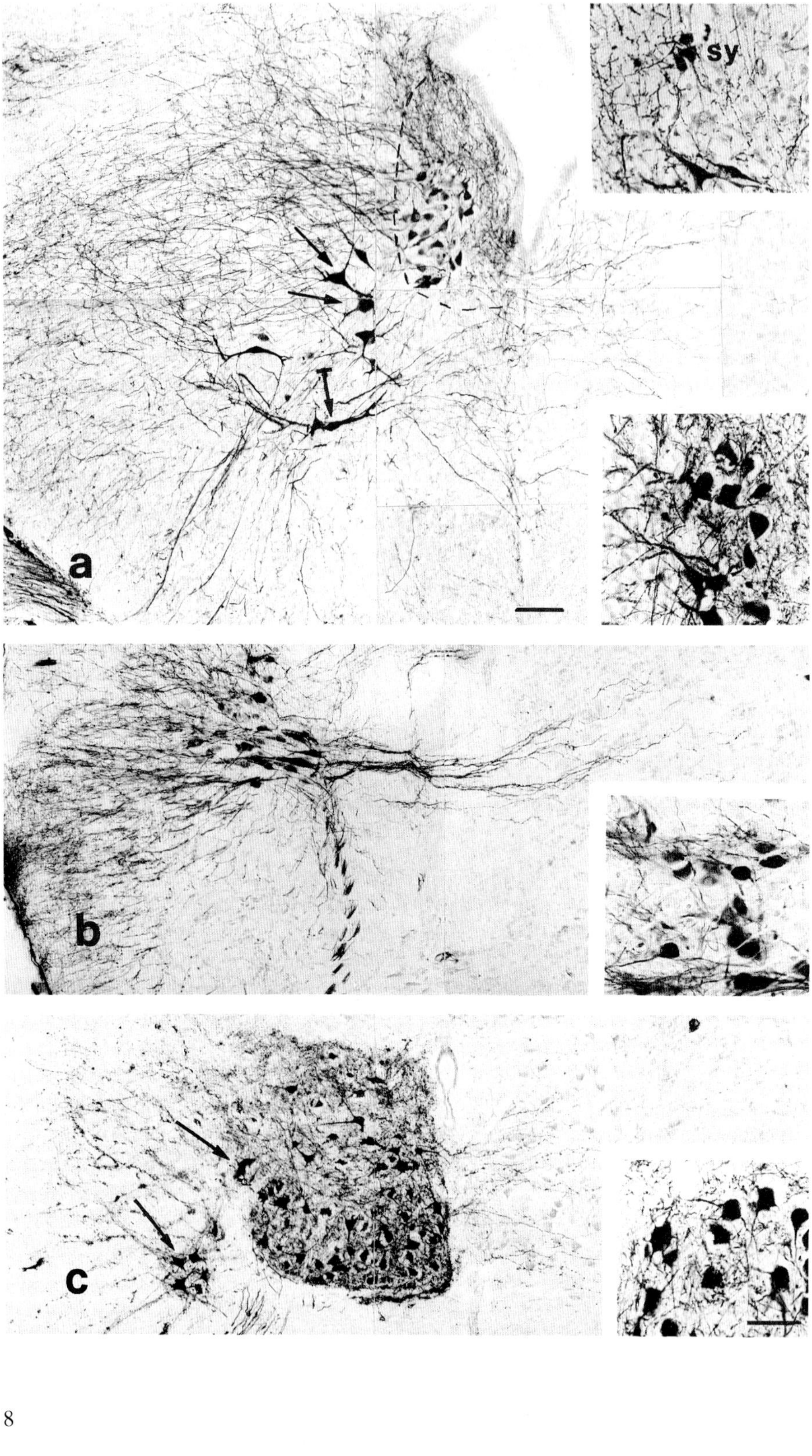
sy
a
b
c

the perikarya. The dorsal dendrites form a dense subependymal plexus and extend dorsally as far as the solitary tract. A significant contingent of their branches crosses to the contralateral side. The ventrolateral dendrites extensively arborize in the white matter covering the area between the motor root and the spinal tract of the trigeminal nerve. The axons originate from the ventrolateral dendritic stem, descend to the caudal pole of the nucleus, and unite with the axons of spinal motoneurons to form the first motor root.

The lateral hypoglossal nucleus begins in the closed part of the medulla and extends beyond the second spinal cord segment. The polygonal perikarya, 40–45 μm in diameter, conspicuously differ, both in form and size, from the neurons of the dorsomedial nucleus (Fig. 1a). The dendrites arborize in all directions, a few branches can be followed to the contralateral side. The axons converge on the exit site of the first spinal nerve.

In urodeles, the hypoglossal nucleus consists also of a dorsomedial and a lateral neuron group. Neurons in the dorsomedial group are almost the exact counterparts of those in the frog: they have a spindle-shaped body and many of them send a strong dendrite to the contralateral side (Wake et al. 1988). Neurons in the lateral group, which seem to be intermingled with other spinal motoneurons, have large oval-shaped perikarya and ipsi- and contralateral dendrite branches. Plethodontine salamanders, which feed by projecting a sticky tongue, have a special neural apparatus for the control of tongue projection in the rostral part of the spinal cord (Roth and Wake 1984, 1985).

3.2 Lizard

The hypoglossal nerve emerges with distinct rootlets from the ventral aspect of the medullospinal junction. It leaves the skull together with the vagal nerve in a common connective tissue sheath and is joined by the combined trunk of the first three spinal nerves. The hypoglossal nucleus consists of a dorsomedial and a ventrolateral neuron group in some reptiles (turtles, crocodilians), and other species (snakes, some lizards) exhibit only one nucleus (see Barbas-Henry and Lohman 1984).

If cobalt is applied to the rootlets of the hypoglossal nerve inside the cranial cavity, a dorsomedial group of neurons is revealed in the obex region (Fig. 1b). The nucleus preserves its dorsomedial position along its rostrocaudal extent and does not merge with other motor nuclei as it terminates in the upper part of the spinal cord (Fig. 18b). The form of neurons closely resembles the frog dorsomedial hypoglossal neurons. They are fusiform or spindle-shaped

◁ **Fig. 1a–c.** The hypoglossal nucleus (photomontages). **a** Frog, obex region. *Broken line* demarcates the hypoglossal nucleus proper, *arrows* point at nerve cells innervating external tongue muscles, and *arrow with bar* indicates spinal motoneurons of trunk muscles. In the *inset* at the *right upper corner* preganglionic sympathetic neurons (sy) are shown. **b** Lizard, obex region. **c** Rat, slightly caudal to the obex. *Arrows* point at motoneurons of external tongue muscles. Note the strong contralateral projections of dendrite bundles of neurons of intrinsic tongue muscles in all cases. Perikarya of these neurons are shown with higher power in the *right lower corners*. *Calibration bar* is 100 μm; 50 μm in the insets and the dendrites arise from the pointed ends of perikarya. The lateral dendrite group expands in a fan-like manner and the terminal twigs reach the subpial zone. Another group of dendrites takes a dorsal course and the branches extend into the subependymal zone. The medial dendrite group crosses to the contralateral side and arborizes in the subependymal zone and in the region of the contralateral hypoglossal nucleus. The axon originates in the medial dendrite stem and turns ventrally toward the site of nerve exit.

Horseradish peroxidase (HRP) application to the hypoglossal nerve outside the cranial cavity reveals a ventrolateral neuron group in the anole as well (Barbas-Henry and Lohman 1988). The ventrolateral neurons are distinctly different from the dorsomedial neurons. They have polygonal large perikarya and radially oriented dendrites which do not cross the midline. Apparently, the ventrolateral neurons innervate the hyoid muscle group.

3.3 Rat

The hypoglossal nerve divides into a lateral and a medial branch in the periphery. If the common nerve trunk is treated with HRP (Krammer et al. 1979) or with cobalt (Matesz 1983), the entire nuclear complex is revealed. It begins in the upper obex region and the tapering end can be followed to the caudal part of the medulla where the pyramidal decussation is completed. Cobalt labeling reveals a small and oval-shaped, and a large and polygonal neuron type (Fig. 1c). Small neurons occupy a dorsomedial position whereas large neurons are found in a lateral position.

The small-celled component form a continuous column along the rostrocaudal extent of the nucleus (Fig. 18c). This cell group lies under the floor of the fourth ventricle in the open part and at the ventral aspect of the central canal in the closed part of the medulla. A septum containing dendritic bundles vaguely separates this subnucleus into a dorsal and a ventral part. The perikarya are oval-shaped or triangular, 22–28 µm in the longer diameter. A lateral and a medial dendritic array emerge from the perikarya. They arborize in a similar manner as described for the lizard. The axon originates from the ventromedial aspect of the cell body and runs straight to the site of exit.

The large-celled component appears in the rostral one third of the nucleus. The size of the perikarya varies between 55 and 45 µm in diameter. The rostrally lying large cells intermingle with the small ones in the lateral part of the nucleus (Fig. 1c). After a short gap, the large cells reappear and form a separate group at the ventrolateral aspect of the nucleus. The dendrites of large cells radiate in all directions, but the medial dendrites abut on the midline. The axons take a straight ventral course toward the site of exit of the small cell axons.

A (dorso-) medial small-celled and a (ventro-) lateral large-celled subdivision can be found in a number of other mammalian species (cat: Miyazaki et al. 1981; dog: Chibuzo and Cummings 1982; monkey: Uemura-Sumi et al. 1981). The somatotopic organization of the hypoglossal nuclear complex is comparable in all these animal species. The small neurons innervate intrinsic tongue muscles. The genioglossus is supplied partly by small cells and partly by large cells from the entire rostrocaudal extent of the nucleus. The styloglossus and hyoglossus receive large cell innervation from the rostral half and the geniohyoideus from the caudal half of the nucleus. The genioglossus receives a bilateral innervation, but the crossing of motor fibers occurs peripherally rather than centrally (Chibuzo and Cummings 1982). In a general trend, intrinsic tongue muscles and the protractor genioglossus are represented in the medial part (small cells), retractors in the lateral part (large cells) of the nucleus.

3.4 Conclusion

From the results presented we conclude that neurons which innervate intrinsic tongue muscles are very similar in their shape and size in frog, lizard and rat (see insets in Fig. 1a,b,c). Their common characteristics are the oval-shaped body, the almost bipolar orientation of the dendritic tree, the crossing medial dendrites, and the ventromedial origin of their axons. No other motoneurons in the medulla and in the upper spinal cord resemble these neurons. The old suggestion that the small-celled part of the hypoglossal nucleus evolved from the rostral part of the spinal motor column seems to be rather improbable. It is more likely that this part of the hypoglossal nucleus is a novel structure of the medulla which appeared concurrently with the acquisition of the muscular tongue during phylogenesis. The large-celled part, however, may represent the "ancient" spino-occipital nucleus which innervates some of the hyoid muscles.

4 The Control of Patterned Eye Movements: The Oculomotor, Trochlear, and Abducens Nuclei

Patterned eye movements, including movements evoked by vestibular and visual stimuli, saccadic eye movements and visual fixation, are performed by the six external eye muscles, four recti and two obliqui, and their activities are controlled by three cranial nerve nuclei from the most primitive cyclostome through primates.

There are some differences in the position and innervation of individual muscles especially in fishes with lateral eyes, and the reader is referred to the literature for the exciting phylogenetic and functional problems related to the differences (Graf and Brunker 1984; Fritzsch et al. 1990). Here, we only want to show the morphology of motoneurons involved in eye movements in the three species investigated.

4.1 The Positions of the Eye Moving Nuclei and the Organization of Muscle Innervation

The familiar dorsomedial positions of these nuclei under the ependyma of the brain stem are consistently described in a large number of different species (Ariëns Kappers et al. 1936; Starck 1982). They are in close topographical, as well as functional, relation to the medial longitudinal fasciculus (mlf). The oculomotor (nIII) and trochlear (nIV) nuclei almost completely fill the longitudinal extent of the mesencephalic central gray matter. These two nuclei are continuous or overlapping in most species, although the nIV can be clearly distinguished. The abducens nucleus (nVI) is in the caudal part of the pontine tegmentum at a level between the caudal pole of the trigeminal and rostral pole of the facial motor nuclei (Fig. 12). Most tetrapods, and some fishes, have an accessory abducens nucleus which will be discussed in Chap. 5.

The organization of muscle innervation is again amazingly uniform from teleost fishes through primates. The general scheme is that the ipsilateral nIII innervates the medial rectus (MR), the inferior rectus (IR), and the inferior obliquus (I0) muscles, whereas the superior rectus (SR) is supplied by the contralateral nucleus. A small ipsilateral component in the innervation of the SR is described in the rat (Labanderia et al. 1983) and the lizard (Barbas-Henry and Lohman 1988). The superior obliquus (SO) receives contralateral innervation from the nIV, although 2%–4% ipsilateral innervation is found in many species (lamprey: Fritzsch et al. 1990; carp: Luiten and Dijkstra-de Vlieger 1978; rodents and carnivores: Murphy et al. 1986). The lateral rectus muscle (LR) is innervated by the ipsilateral nVI.

The fine somatotopic representation of individual muscles within the nIII is also described for a large number of different species. The general tendency is that motoneurons innervating the MR muscle are located dorsomedially but with a differential distribution along the rostrocaudal axis. The IR muscle is represented in the dorsolateral region with partial overlap with the MR. The I0 is innervated mainly from the ventrolateral part of the ipsilateral nucleus, the SO from the ventromedial part of the contralateral nucleus mainly from its caudal pole. This spatial segregation of motoneurons is clearest in the chick (Heaton and Wayne 1983) and the monkey (Porter et al. 1983). Differences in minor details, especially in the localization of I0 and SR motoneurons, are found in guinea pigs and rabbits (Evinger et al. 1987; Murphy et al. 1986). There are overlaps to various extents between the areas of representation in fishes (Szabo et al. 1987) and in frogs (Matesz and Székely 1977). No clear segregation of motoneurons is evident in salamanders (Naujoks-Manteuffel et al. 1986) and in rats (Labanderia et al. 1983). There are some deviations from this general scheme of innervation in primitive fishes (Graf and Brunker 1984; Fritzsch et al. 1990).

4.2 Neuronal Morphology in the Eye Moving Nuclei

4.2.1 Frog

In neurons labeled with cobalt, the eye moving nuclei are oval-shaped with polygonal perikarya (Matesz and Székely 1977). The cell body is relatively small, 17–25 μm at the longest diameter; that is, it is about two thirds the size of a hypoglossal cell body. Although there are some common features in the morphology of neurons, the dendritic tree spreads differently in the three nuclei. This may be due to structural differences in their environment.

In the nIII the dendritic tree expands extensively in a fan-like manner and covers a semicircular area which extends from the floor of the mesencephalic aqueduct to the interpeduncular nucleus (Fig. 2a). Within the fan-like arborization pattern, a dorsomedial–ventrolateral direction can be distinguished in the orientation of the main dendritic branches. A rostral extension of dendrites reaches the caudal one third of the diencephalon, and a compact narrow bundle stretches caudally among the neurons of the nIV. A similar pattern of arborization can be seen in the nVI with the exception that the secondary and tertiary branches of dorsomedial and ventrolaertal dendrites are separated by the intervening gray matter of the pontine tegmentum (Figs. 3d, 4a). In the nIV, the enlarged posteroventral tegmental nucleus pushes the dorsomedial dendrites in the lateral direction and the increasingly large mlf separates them from the ventrolateral dendrites. The two dendritic groups hug, as it were, the mlf. Crossing dendrites are not presented by any of these nuclei.

The axon, as a rule, originates from one of the ventrolaterally directed main dendrites. There are two exceptions to this rule. First, the crossing oculomotor axons which emerge from a dorsomedial dendrite, cross the midline, turn about the dorsolateral aspect of the contralateral nucleus and join the ipsilateral axon bundle (Fig. 2a). The second exception is the course of

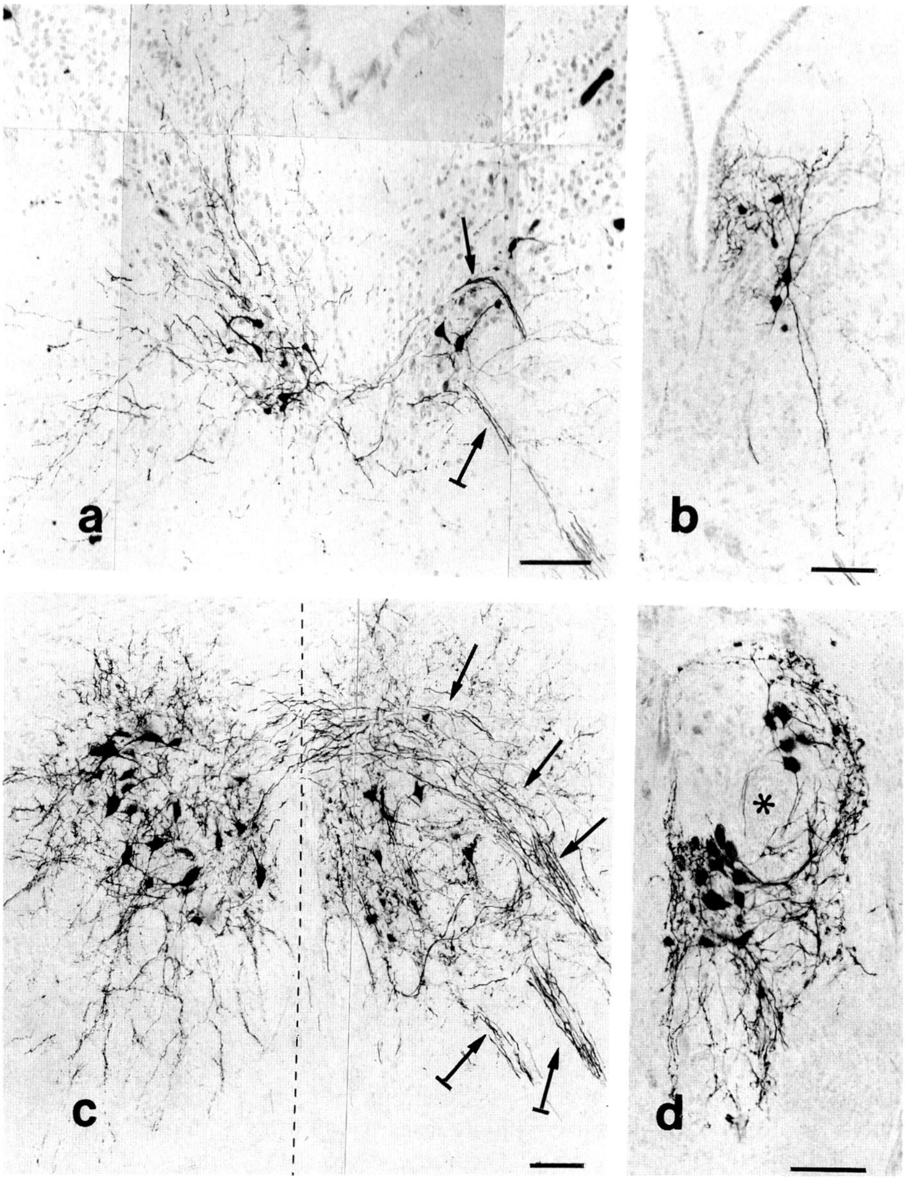

Fig. 2a–d. The oculomotor nucleus. The right oculomotor nerve was filled with cobalt in each case. **a** Frog, (photomontage). The *arrow* points at the bend of crossing axons, *arrow with bar* indicates ipsilateral axons. **b**, **d** Lizard; in **b** the rostral pole, in **d** the caudal part of the nucleus is shown. *Asterisk* shows the medial longitudinal fasciculus. **c** Rat (photomontage). *Arrows* indicate the arched course of crossing axons, *arrows with bar* point at ipsilateral axons. The *broken line* is on the midline. *Calibration bar* is 100 μm

trochlear axons. They originate in a laterally directed dendrite, travel along the lateral border of the gray matter, pierce the velum medullare, and emerge on the contralateral side (Fig. 3a).

4.2.2 Lizard

In view of the thick dendritic tangle obtained from cobalt labeling, it is not possible to give a similar detailed description of the dendritic arborization pattern in the lizard (Székely and Matesz 1988). The perikarya are oval-shaped or polygonal, 11–14 μm at the longer diameter. They are conspicuously smaller than the hypoglossal neurons. At the rostral pole of the nucleus, a dorsomedial and a ventrolateral dendrite group can be recognized (Fig. 2b), but more caudally these dendrites hug the medial and lateral aspects of the nucleus in the center of which the mlf is formed (Fig. 2d). The ipsilateral axons originate in the ventrolateral aspect of the soma and take a straight course to the site of exit. Axons innervating the contralateral SR can be followed, over consecutive sections, to the dorsal aspect of the contralateral nIII, where they sharply turn in the ventral direction to enter the oculomotor root on the contralateral side.

The nIV is the continuation of the dorsolateral subnucleus overlapping the contralateral oculomotor neurons. The dendrites form a medial and a lateral arm which border the caudal pole of the nIII. The axons emerge from the dorsolateral aspect of the somata and cross in the velum medullare (Fig. 3b). The perikarya in the nVI are similar to those in the above mentioned nuclei (Figs. 3e, 4c). They are situated at the ventrolateral aspect of the mlf. A dorsal dendrite group extends to the floor of the 4th ventricle, and the ventrolateral group extends in the direction of the accessory abducens nucleus. The axon arises from the ventral part of the cell body.

4.2.3 Rat

In addition to a few oval-shaped perikarya, polygonal cell bodies dominate in the rat nIII (Fig. 2c). Their size varies to a greater extent than in frogs or in lizards, measuring 16–26 μm in the longer diameter. The dendrites radiate out apparently in all directions, but the medial branches abut on the midline and form a demarcating dendrite plexus at the medial aspect of the nucleus. In the dorsal, lateral, and ventral directions they cover a semicircular area resembling very much the arborization pattern seen in the frog. The ipsilateral axons originate in the ventral part, the crossing axons in the dorsal part of the somata. These latter axons pass round the contralateral nucleus with a sharp bend (Fig. 2c).

There is a gap of about 100 μm between the nIII and the nIV. The trochlear nucleus is a globular body extending about 250 μm caudally. It contains the same types of neurons as seen in the nIII. The axon arises from the ventral aspects of the cell body and after a short initial ventral course it sharply turns in the dorsolateral direction follows the lateral border of the

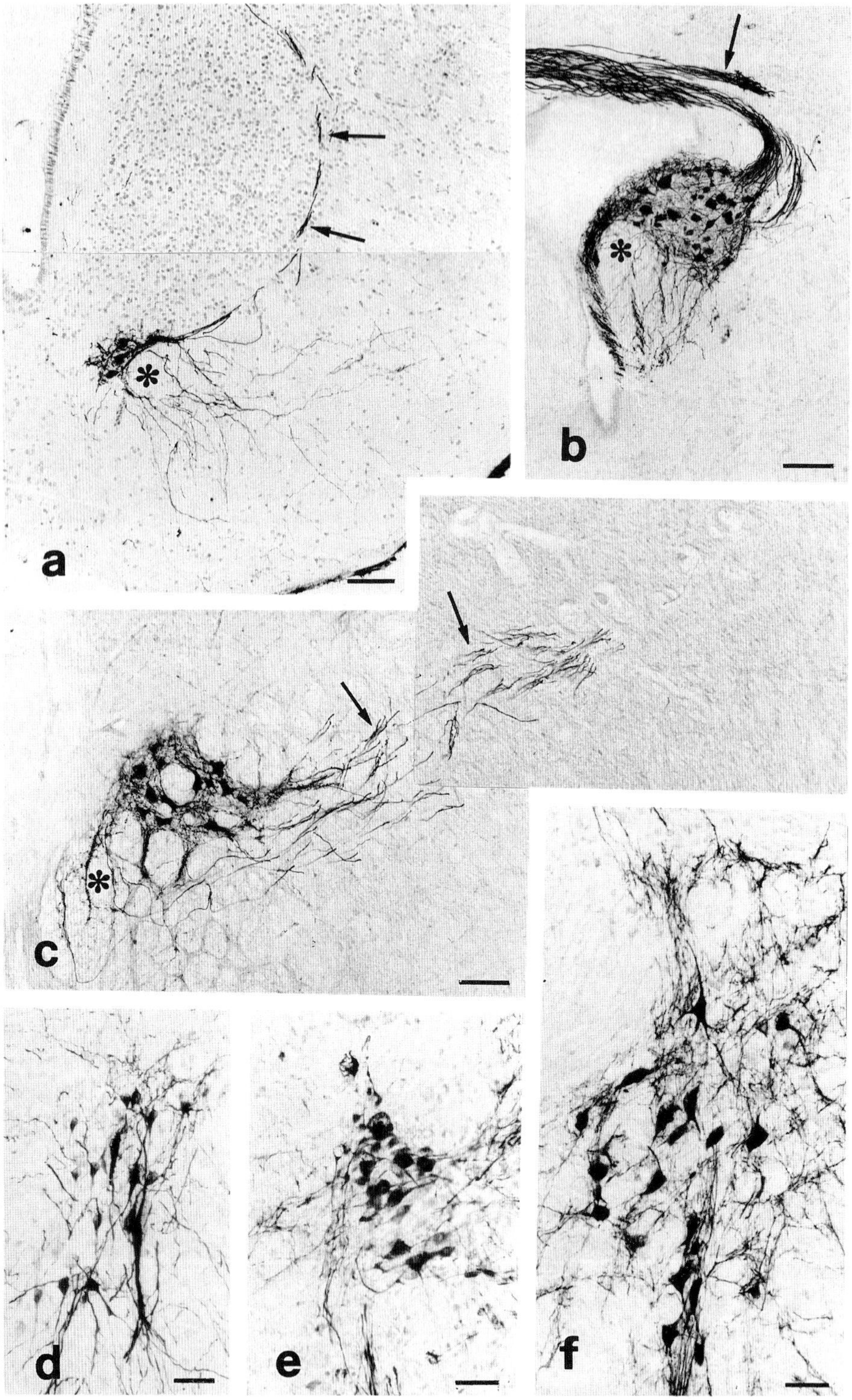
a
b
c
d
e
f

central gray substance, and runs in the direction of the anterior medullare velum (Fig. 3c).

The nVI is squeezed in between the mlf and the facial genu (Fig. 4e). The cell body is elongated, polygonal and measures about 20 µm in the longer diameter (Fig. 3f). The "squeezed in" position apparently determines the pattern of dendritic arborization. Strong dendrite branches extend dorsally as far as the floor of the fourth ventricle. A number of medially directed dendrites penetrate the mlf, while lateral dendrites abut on the facial genu. The axon emerges from the ventral aspect of the cell body.

4.3 Conclusion

Taking into account the size and shape of perikarya, the pattern of dendritic arborization, and the origin and course of axons, there are distinct differences between hypoglossal and eye moving motoneurons. The dorsomedial nuclear column is, therefore, composed of characteristically different forms of neurons. Although the interspecies similarities are not as clear in the eye moving nuclei as in the nXII, still the morphology of eye moving neurons has a closer resemblance across the three species investigated than does the morphology of the hypoglossal and eye moving neurons in the same species.

As mentioned earlier, the dorsomedial motor column is also called the somatomotor column. This terminology is adapted from the development of intrinsic tongue muscles from the segmented occipital mesoderm which is homologous with the segmented mesoderm in the trunk region. Since trunk segments give rise to somatic muscles, tongue muscles originating from occipital muscles should be somatic muscles. Their motor nucleus (the nXII) is, therefore, a somatomotor nucleus which is in one dorsomedial line with the eye moving motor nuclei forming the common somatomotor column. Consequently, the external eye muscles are somatic muscles and they should have derived also from the segmented mesoderm. This implicit reasoning is one of the basic arguments in favor of the existence of preotic head segments in the old literature. However, there is not a uniform somatomotor column, as far as the morphology of the component neurons is concerned, and there is no reason to classify eye muscles and tongue muscles into one common somatic muscle group with an assumption of their common origin. This question will be discussed later.

The crossing oculomotor axons take a distinct ventral turn at the dorsolateral aspect of the nIII in frogs, lizard, and rats. It is generally believed that neurons with crossing axons migrate across the midline during development, and the path of migration is indicated by the trajectory of axons. According to this assumption, these neuroblasts ought to have migrated along this devious route

◁ **Fig. 3a–f.** The trochlear (**a**, **b**, **c**,) and the abducens (**d**, **e**, **f**,) nuclei. **a** Frog (photomontage); **b** lizard; **c** rat (photomontage). In each figure *arrows* point at the crossing axon bundle and the *asterisk* is in the medial longitudinal fasciculus. **d**, **e**, **f** The abducens nucleus of the frog, lizard, and rat, respectively. Note the similar form of the perikarya. *Calibration bar* is 100 µm in **a**, **b**, and **c**; 50 µm in **d**, **e**, and **f** cruising about the nucleus and arriving at its ventrolateral part (see Figs. 2a,c). This does not seem very probable, and it has been recently shown that, in the *Xenopus* toad, neurons with crossing axons differentiate in the contralateral side, the axon decussates very early in the embryo, and the neurons migrate to a medial position on the side of their origin much later in development (Matesz 1990b). This explains the curious ventral bend of the contralateral oculomotor axons. The decussation and the dorsal exit of the trochlear nerve remain an enigma. At this point one may think of the extreme dorsal position of the nIV in the lamprey (Fig. 1B of Fritzsch et al. 1990). From this position, the outgrowing axons might have an easier access to the dorsal surface, and as the group of neurons may have shifted ventrally during phylogenesis, the trajectory of trochlear axons indicates this secondary migration.

5 The Protection of the Eye: The Accessory Abducens Nucleus

In addition to the six external eye muscles, tetrapods have an additional set of muscles, the retractor bulbi (Nishi 1938). It usually consists of four slips of muscle which surround the optic nerve within the space of the cone of the six external eye muscles and insert behind the equator of the eye bulb. They withdraw the eye into the orbit and this allows the nictitating membrane to slide over the eye, thereby protecting and lubricating the cornea. In birds, this muscle group is found in the form of the pyramidal and quadrate muscles which inserts on the nictitating membrane and moves it actively. Chiroptera and primates do not have this muscle group. The retractor bulbi, pyramidal, and quadrate muscles are innervated by the abducens nerve, and the innervating fibers originate in the accessory abducens nucleus (nVIa).

5.1 The Position of the Accessory Abducens Nucleus

The nucleus was recognized by van Gehuchten (1898a) in birds, its significance and comparative anatomy was studied by Addens (1933). It lies at the level between the trigeminal and facial motor nuclei in the magnocellular part of the reticular formation and is often mistaken for these cells in the old descriptions. The nucleus can be only identified by showing the characteristic trajectory of its axons. The neurons are situated ventrolateral and slightly caudal to the main abducens nucleus (Figs. 12, 18). The rostral pole of the accessory abducens nucleus coincides with the caudal pole of the main nucleus. It is present in all tetrapods investigated with modern tracing techniques (Urodeles: Naujoks-Manteuffel et al. 1986; frog: Matesz and Székely 1977; bird: Heaton and Wayne 1983; lizard: Székely and Matesz 1988; rat: Székely and Matesz 1982; rabbit and guinea pig: Evinger et al. 1987; cat: Spencer et al. 1980).

5.2 The Neuronal Morphology in the Accessory Abducens Nucleus

With the cobalt labeling technique, the shape and dendritic arborization pattern in the frog, lizard, and rat are so similar that we can describe them here together. The longitudinally extended polygonal perikaryon is characteristic of all three species (Fig. 4b,d,f). The long axis of the soma is in the dorsomedial-ventrolateral direction and measures 35–45 µm; the neurons are, therefore, considerably larger than those in the main nVI. The ventrolateral dendrite group very characteristically forms a compact broom-like bundle from which a

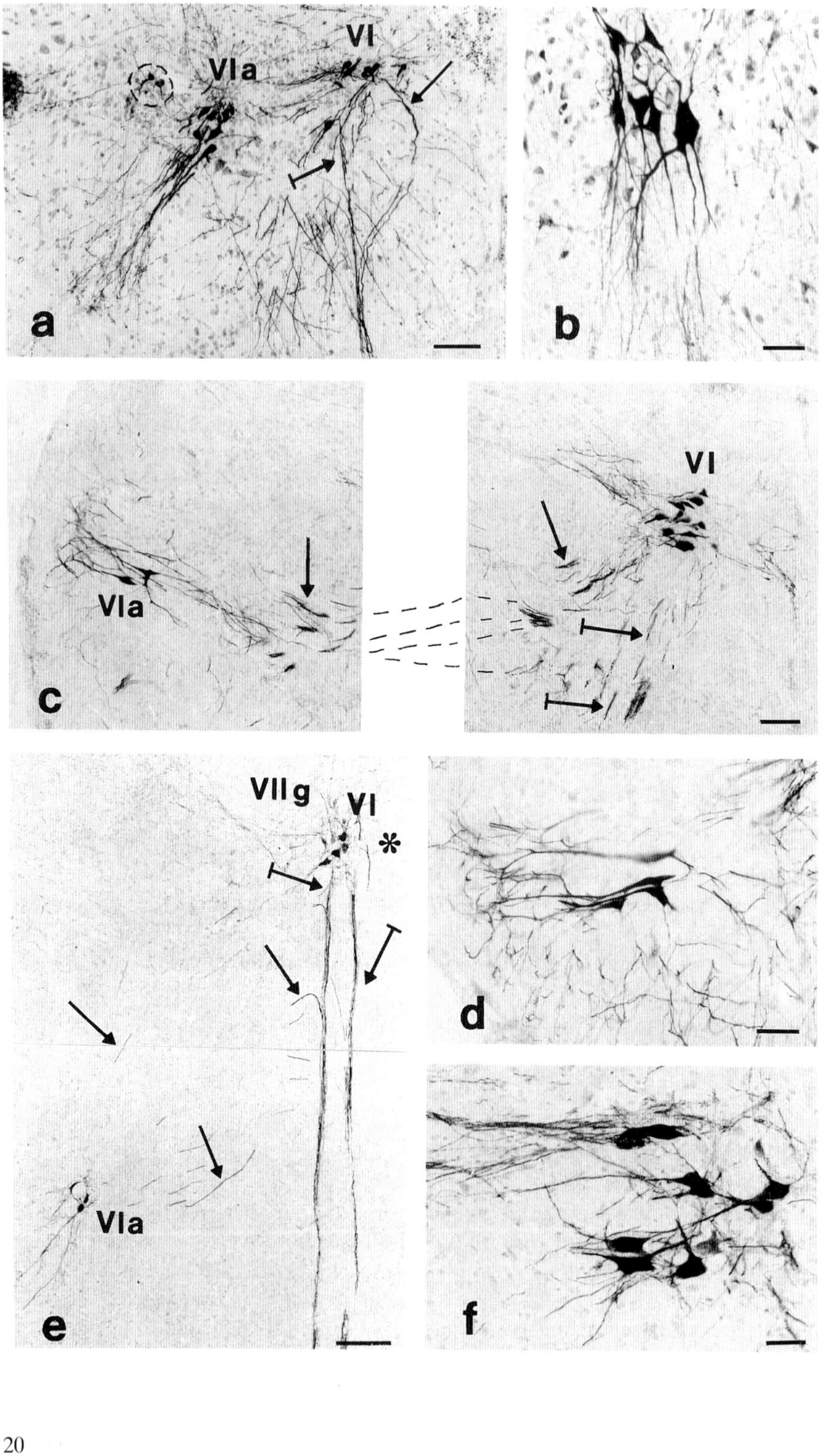

VI
VIa
a
b
VIa
c
VI
VIIg
VI
*
VIa
e
d
f

few branches extend into the nucleus of the spinal tract of the trigeminal nerve (nspV). The dorsomedial dendrite group is labeled less successfully; it spreads in a fan-like manner in the reticular formation. The axon originates in the dorsomedial aspect of the perikaryon, or in one of the dorsomedial dendrites, runs in the dorsomedial direction and, upon reaching the main nucleus, sharply turns in the ventral direction to join the abducens fibers (Figs. 4a,c,e). Neurons with very similar morphology are described in the nVIa of salamanders with HRP labeling of the nerve (Naujoks-Manteuffel et al. 1986) and in the cat with intramuscular HRP injection (Spencer et al. 1980).

5.3 The Function of the Accessorius Abducens – Retractor Bulbi System

The position of the nVIa, away from the mlf and close to the nspV, suggests that the nucleus' main source of afferentation is the trigeminal system. It has been shown in the cat by Baker et al. (1980) that electrical stimulation of the ophthalmic and maxillary nerves, and of the ipsilateral and contralateral cornea, evoked large amplitude disynaptic excitatory postsynaptic potentials. Neurons in the other external eye muscle nuclei did not usually respond with similar short latency activation to these stimuli. The powerful vestibular effect known to be present in other eye muscle motor nuclei (Baker and Highstein 1978) was not observed in the nVIa neurons; rather, they showed a weak disynaptic ipsilateral inhibition. These findings are consistent with previous suggestions, that the nVIa is a unique neural structure for controlling eye withdrawal.

While the nVIa seems to innervate exclusively the retractor muscles they receive innervation from other sources as well. By gross dissection, Murphy et al. (1986) found oculomotor nerve branches entering the retractor bulbi in the rabbit, and Gray et al. (1981) could label nVI neurons by injecting HRP into the retractor bulbi of the rabbit. This pattern of innervation suggests that the retractor muscles also take part in patterned eye movements.

The close relation of the nVIa with the nspV and the common exit of its axons with nVI axons provided the basis for the idea of neurobiotaxis (Ariëns Kappers et al. 1936). This idea maintains that the presumptive nVIa neuroblasts migrate from the nVI primordium in order to settle in the vicinity of their primary source of afferentation, that is the nspV. This suggestion has been generalized to explain various cell migrations during development. The conspicuous morphological and functional differences between nVIa and nVI neurons do not support the assumption that these neurons are derived from a

◁ **Fig. 4a–f.** The accessory abducens nucleus. In each figure *VI* and *VIa* indicate the main and the accessory abducens nuclei, respectively. *Arrows* point at the axons of VIa neurons and *arrows with bar* at the axons of VI neurons. **a**, **b** Frog. In **a**, the cell group demarcated by the *broken line* represents parasympathetic preganglionic neurons of Harder's gland. **c**, **d** Lizard; the two sides of **c** are taken from different levels. **e**, **f** Rat; in **e** *VIIg* indicates the internal genu of the facial nerve, and the *asterisk* is in the medial longitudinal fasciculus. Note the similarity of the shape of VIa neurons in **b**, **d**, **f**. *Calibration bar* is 50 μm in **b**, **d**, **f**; 100 μm in **a**, **c**; 200 μm in **e** common primordium. Furthermore, in a recent HRP and cobalt labeling study, Matesz (1990a) succeeded in showing that: (a) nVIa neuroblasts differentiated laterally to the nVI primordium, (b) they were much bigger than the nVI neuroblasts, and (c) they distinctly differed from them in shape.

5.4 Conclusion

From the neuronal morphology and synaptic convectivity of nVIa motoneurons it appears that a special apparatus has evolved for the protection of the eye and the lubrication of the cornea in tetrapods. The appearance of this apparatus coincides with the ability for, and is the condition of, land life. Both periphery and center seem to be novel structures differentiated in phylogenesis for a special function. Curiously, this apparatus is not found in primates. Fritzsch et al. (1990) describe a group of motoneurons in the ventrolateral part of the pontine tegmentum which innervates the caudal rectus muscle in the lamprey. Since this cell group is at the level of the nVI and its position is reminiscent of the nVIa in tetrapods, they suggest homology between these ventral neurons and the caudal rectus and the nVIa and the retractor bulbi muscles. There are a number of problems with this homology. First, in the lamprey, the nIII innervates three muscles and the nVI two muscles, which is a unique pattern in vertebrates. Second, the assumed nVIa of the lamprey innervates one of the six extraocular muscles which controls patterned movements. (What would be the advantage if a lamprey could retract its eyes?) Third, it is known that motor cells of extraocular muscles are poorly segregated in fish, especially the cells of the abducens (Szabo et al. 1987). The poor segregation is also found in the lamprey, in which nIV and nVI neurons are dispersed over a wide area (see Fig. 1 of Fritzsch et al. 1990). Fourth, no trace of a ventrolateral abducens neuron group can be seen in higher fishes. Could it be that the primordium of the nVIa – retractor bulbi system is present in the most primitive vertebrate having eyes, and that it disappears and reappears again in tetrapods? Some teleosts also have two abducens nuclei, one rostral and one caudal (Sterling 1977), and they innervate the caudal (lateral) rectus muscle. The rostral part of the muscle contains tonic muscle fibers, the caudal part contains phasic muscle fibers (Gestrin and Sterling 1977). The two nuclei represent a tonic-phasic spatial distribution which may be present in other nuclei as well, although without spatial segregation.

In the monkey, there is an accessory lateral rectus muscle which is held to be homologous with the lateral slip of the retractor bulbi muscle and a few ventrally disposed abducens motoneurons are regarded as the nVIa by Schnyder (1984). However, as has been correctly pointed out by Spencer and Porter (1981), unlike the nVIa neurons, these ventral abducens neurons innervate both the lateral rectus and the accessory lateral rectus muscles and intermingle with the dorsal abducens neurons. Furthermore, they are at the rostral rather than at the caudal pole of the main VI nucleus. Furthermore the accessory lateral rectus muscle resemble the lateral rectus muscle both structurally and functionally. They speculate that with the deep bony orbit the retractor bulbi muscles lost their significance.

The corneal reflex remains an enigma in human. When simply blinking the eyelid is dropped by the relaxed levator palpebrae. A strong "corneal reflex" is achieved by the contraction of the orbicularis oculi muscle innervated by the facial nerve.

6 Control of Jaw Movements and Facial Expression: The Trigeminal and Facial Nuclei

The description of these two nuclei together is motivated by their joint activity in the control of the primary mandibular joint. The secondary (mammalian) mandibular joint is controlled only by the trigeminal nerve. A part of the structural transformation which results in the secondary jaw joint is the appearance of muscles for mastication and facial expression. Concurrent with the transformation of the periphery, profound structural changes occur in the center and these changes are rather equivocally treated in the literature. We think that the joint discussion of these two motor nuclei from a functional point of view promotes the understanding of species differences in these nuclei. In this effort, we give a short overview of the evolution of the primary and secondary mandibular joints and their muscles before describing the corresponding motor centers.

6.1 The Primary Mandibular Joint and Its Muscles

This type of joint is present in amphibians, generalized reptiles, and birds. It is also called the articular-quadrate joint, as it is formed between a posterior extension (the articular) of the dentary bone (the primary mandible) and an inferior process (the quadrate) of the palatoquadrate bone. The joint acts as the hinge of a two-armed lever (Fig. 5a) and the structural restriction permits only opening and closing of the mouth. Animals with the primary mandibular joint can only grasp and swallow food but they cannot chew and grind it.

Muscles associated with the articular-quadrate joint are derived from an originally uniform primordial constrictor muscle (Starck 1982). In the region of the first branchial arch, the middle part of the constrictor muscle gives rise to the adductor mandibulae from which a complex set of muscles differentiates for the closing of the mouth. The ventral part of the constrictor provides the intermandibularis muscle which forms the floor of the mouth. These muscles are innervated by the mandibular nerve of the trigeminus. In the region of the second branchial arch, the constrictor splits into a deep and a superficial sheet. The deep sheet gives rise to the interhyoideus and the depressor mandibulae muscles. The former merges with the intermandibularis and contributes to the muscular floor of the mouth muscles. The latter inserts on a posterior extension of the articulare and opens the mouth. The superficial sheet forms the sphincter colli. These muscles are innervated by the facial nerve.

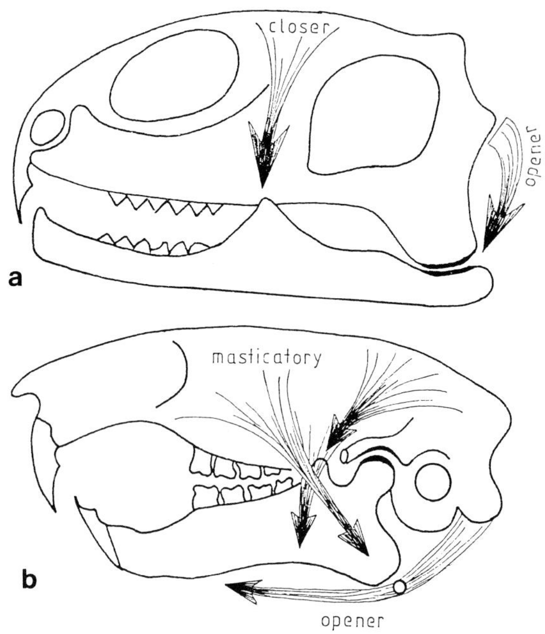

Fig. 5a,b. The primary and secondary mandibular joints. *Thick lines* indicate articular facets. **a** Articular-quadrate joint of a generalized reptile. *Arrows* show the line of force of the closer and opener muscles. **b** The temporomandibular joint of a mammal (rodent). Note the complex lines of force of the masticatory muscles

6.2 The Secondary Mandibular Joint and Its Muscles

Parallel with a series of complicated transformations (Crompton 1989), the articular-quadrate joint becomes the incudomalleolar joint and the temporomandibular joint evolves in its stead (Fig. 5b). It is the characteristic jaw joint of all mammals. Anatomically, this joint is placed in a more rostral position than the primary mandibular joint, that is, the mandible and its muscles lie in the region of the trigeminal nerve. The structure of the joint and the position of muscles render possible a variety of movements including opening and closing, lateral translation, and protraction and retraction of the mandible resulting in the masticatory movements characteristic of mammals.

The masticatory muscles are conventionally derived from the same muscle primordium which gives rise to the jaw closing muscles of the primary mandibular joint. However, Starck (1982) observes that the muscle mass undergoes such radical remodeling in reconstruction of the mandibular joint and middle ear region that individual homologization is not possible. The suprahyoid muscles, by contrast, can be homologized with the intermandibularis muscle of the primary mandible. In addition to forming the floor of the mouth, these muscles open the jaw in mammals. All muscles involved in the movement of the secondary mandibular joint are innervated by the mandibular nerve. The deep sheet of the primordial constrictor muscle gives rise to the stapedius, the posterior belly of the digastric and the stylohyoid muscles in the region of the facial nerve.

The superficial sheet, the primitive sphincter colli, is the matrix of the muscles of facial expression (Huber 1930, but see Sect. 6.6).

6.3 The Control of Movements at the Primary Mandibular Joint: The Amphibian and Sauropsidian Trigeminal and Facial Nuclei

6.3.1 Frog

The trigeminal motor nucleus (nV) extends from the level of the cerebellar nuclei to the entrance zone of the statoacoustic nerve in the lateral zone of the pontine gray matter (Matesz and Székely 1978). A neck incompletely separates the caudal pole from the larger rostral part of the nucleus (Fig. 18a). Motoneurons can be divided into three morphologically distinct types. The first consists of large neurons (40–50 μm) with slightly elongated polygonal or star-shaped perikarya (Fig. 6b). The dendritic arbor is arranged in the dorsomedial-ventrolateral direction (Fig. 6c). The slender dorsomedial dendrities arborize in a fan-like manner under the floor of the fourth ventricle, the ventrolateral dendrites form a characteristic broom-like arborization pattern. The axon emerges either from a dendrite stem or from the perikaryon, and after an initial dorsolateral course it turns ventrally toward the root exit. In rare occasions the axon takes a dorsomedial direction and with a hairpin loop turns back toward the motor root (Fig. 6c). With separate labeling of individual branches of the mandibular nerve, it can be shown that this type of motoneurons innervates the jaw closing muscles.

Neurons in the second type are smaller (25–32 μm) and the perikarya are rounded or oval-shaped (Fig. 6d,e, Fig. 10a). The orientation and arborization pattern of dendrites and the course of axons correspond to that described for the first group. These neurons supply the submaxillary and submental (intermandibularis) muscles.

The third type represents a separate class with respect to both the form and innervation area of neurons (Székely and Matesz 1987). The perikaryon is polygonal and is about the same size as that in the second group. The dendrites radiate out in all directions covering about one-half of the brain stem cross-section (Fig. 6a). The axons emerge from the dorsolateral aspect of the perikaryon and join the motor root. In the periphery, they run in the

Fig. 6a–g. The trigeminal and the facial nuclei of the frog. **a** Neurons innervating the levator bulbi muscles. The unstained neurons within the framed area indicate the extent of the nV innervating jaw closer muscles. **b** A motoneuron of the masseter muscle. **c** The rostral part of the nV. The darkly stained area in the *upper left corner* represents sensory fibers of the trigeminal nerve. A *large arrow* indicates the motor root. The *small* and the *large brackets* embrace the extent of arborization of the ventrolateral and dorsomedial dendrites. *Arrows* point at type 1 neurons. The *arrow with bar* shows an axon which forms a medial loop before joining the motor root. **d** The caudal part of the nV. It consists of type 2 neurons. *Arrows* indicate the axons. **e** Two motoneurons of the intermandibularis muscle. **f** The nVII. It consists of type 2 neurons. The *arrow* points at the motor root. **g** A motoneuron of the depressor mandibulae muscle. *Calibration bar* is 100 μm ▷

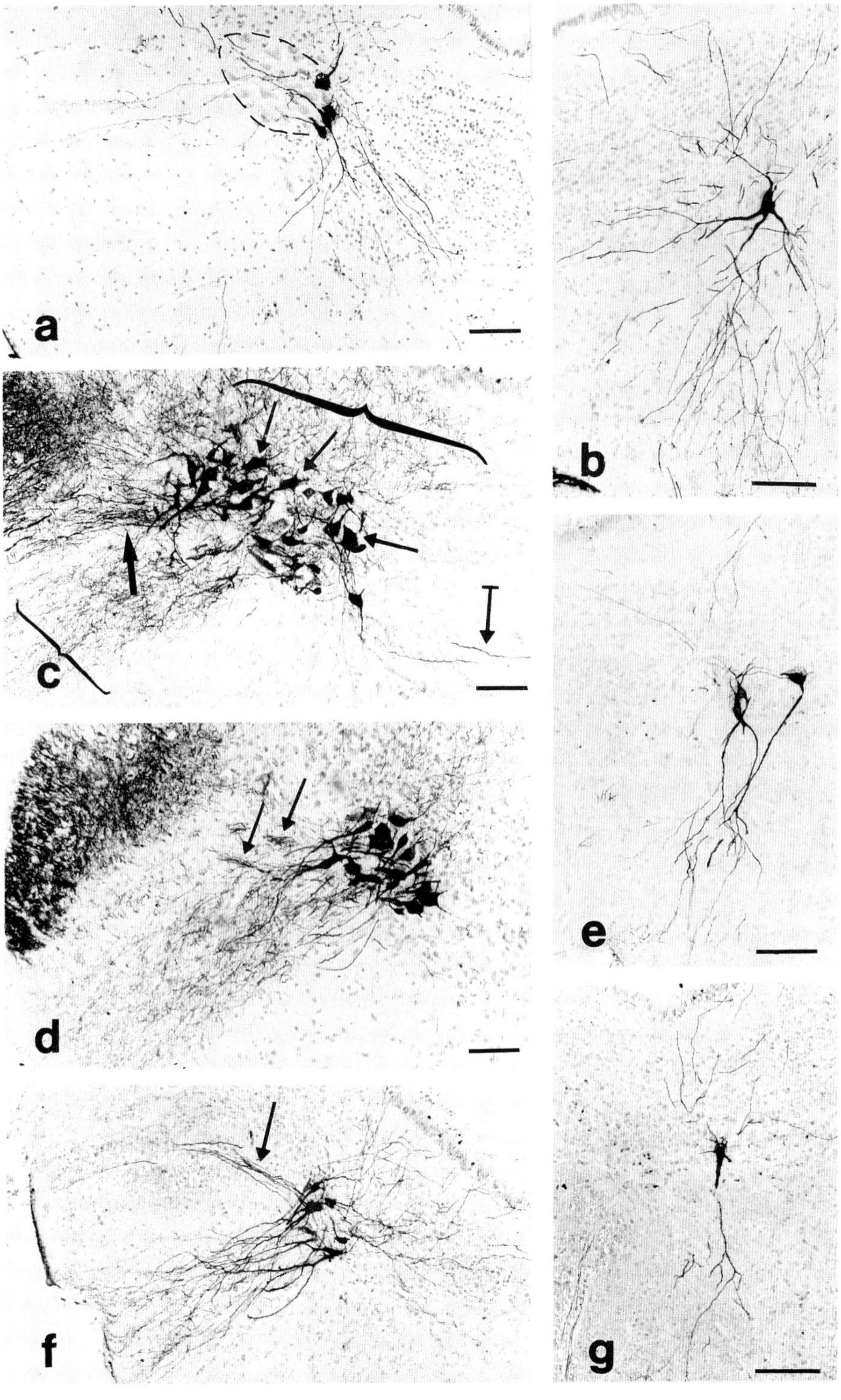

a
b
c
d
e
f
g

Table 1. The long and short diameters of motoneurons innervating the jaw closing (*) and opening (**) muscles in the frog ($n = 20$)

	Long diameter (μm)	Short diameter (μm)
Temporalis*	38.02 ± 8.87	22.11 ± 4.51
Masseter*	45.51 ± 6.48	24.79 ± 6.48
Pterygoid*	50.32 ± 12.38	19.58 ± 4.84
Intermandibularis**	30.45 ± 6.91	18.84 ± 5.19
Depressor mandibulae**	31.51 ± 6.62	17.42 ± 3.91

ophthalmic and maxillary nerves and innervate the levator bulbi, which is a thin sheet of muscle separating the orbit from the oral cavity. This type of neuron and the muscle are present only in amphibians.

The three types of neurons are distributed in a very characteristic manner in the nV (Matesz and Hevessy 1992). The third type is represented only by a few (16–20) neurons and they form a compact group at the dorsomedial aspect of the rostral pole of the nucleus (Fig. 18a). The first type can be found in the larger rostral two thirds of the nucleus. Neurons supplying the temporal, masseter and pterygoid muscles are mixed; however they can be distinguished by their size (Table 1). The tapering caudal one third is constituted solely by the second type of neuron (Fig. 6d).

The facial motor nucleus (nVII) is a well-defined spherical group of motoneurons about 170 μm caudal to the nV in the ventrolateral motor column (Matesz and Székely 1978). The caudal pole extends almost to the level of the nV (Fig. 18a), ventrally it is bordered by the large Mauthner neuron. The nucleus consists of neurons which are the exact counterparts of type 2 neurons in the nV (Figs. 6f,g, 11b, Table 1). They innervate the posterior part of the intermandibularis (interhyoideus) and the depressor mandibulae. Facial neurons, therefore, open the jaw.

6.3.2 Lizard

The organization of the nV and the form of the constituent neurons are more complex in this animal (Székely and Matesz 1988). The rostral pole is at the cerebellar peduncle. Here the nucleus is broad and can be divided into the small-celled dorsomedial and the large-celled ventrolateral subnuclei (Fig. 7a). The dorsomedial part gradually tapers off in the middle of the nucleus; the ventrolateral part terminates at the level of the nVI (Fig. 18b). The orientation and pattern of dendritic arborization are very similar to that described for the frog: the dorsomedial dendrites arborize in a fan-like manner, the ventrolateral dendrites present the broom-like pattern. The trajectory of the axon is a common and very characteristic feature of all types of neurons: it arises from the dorsal part of the neuron, runs dorsomedially or medially sometimes

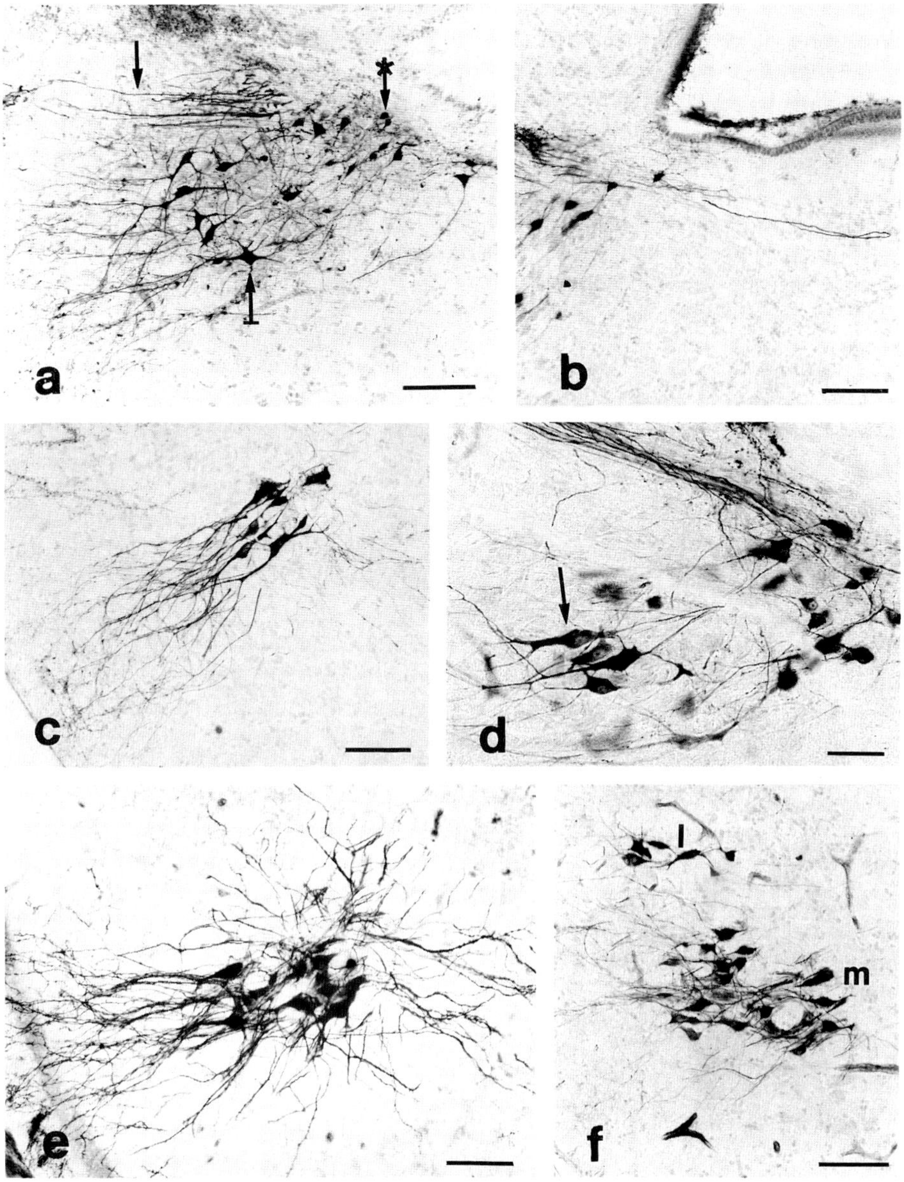

Fig. 7a–f. The trigeminal and facial nuclei of the lizard. **a** The rostral part of the nV. The *arrow with asterisk* shows a type 1 (small) neuron and the *arrow with bar* a polygonal large neuron (type 3). Simple *arrow* shows the motor root. **b** An axon is shown as it forms a medial hairpin turn. **c** The caudal part of the nV. It consists of type 2 neurons. **d** The large variety of spindle-shaped neurons (type 2) are shown (*arrow*) in the middle part of the nV. **e** The rostral part of the nVII. It consists of type 2 neurons. **f** The lateral (*l*) and medial (*m*) subnuclei of the nVII. Calibration bar is 50 μm in **d**; 100 μm in **a–c**, **e**, **f**

reaching the mlf, then turns laterally with a loop, or a hairpin bend, in the direction of the motor root (Fig. 7b).

According to the size and shape of the perikarya, three different types can be distinguished. The first type is represented by small (10–12 μm) neurons with round or oval perikarya which give rise to relatively few dendrites (Fig. 7a). They are located in the dorsomedial part of the nucleus. The second type consists of spindle-shaped neurons which are found throughout the large-celled part of the nucleus and constitute the majority of the cell population. A large (40–50 μm) (Fig. 7d) and a small (20–25 μm) (Fig. 7c, 10c) version can be distinguished in this type of neuron. The third type contains neurons of various forms. The perikaryon may be oval or round, pear- or beet-shaped, or multipolar (Fig. 7a). A large (45–50 μm) and a middle-sized (25–30 μm) variety can be discerned also in this group. Initially the dendrites may take any direction, but the secondary and tertiary branches remain within the confines of the typical broom-like arborization pattern (Fig. 7c).

Application of cobalt to the facial nerve proximal to the geniculate ganglion reveals two well-defined cellular aggregates representing the medial and lateral facial nuclei (Fig. 7e,f). The medial nucleus lies in the same rostrocaudal line with the nV, with a gap of about 1 mm between the two nuclei. The tapering end can be followed almost as far as the closed part of the medulla where the two subnuclei merge as the medial one shifts laterally (Fig. 18b). Two subnuclei of the facial nerve are present in a similar location in the *Varanus* as well (Barbas-Henry 1982). As shall be shown later, the facial and glossopharyngeal nuclei merge in the lizard.

The medial subnucleus consists of the small version of the second type of trigeminal neuron (Figs. 7f, 10d). The axons ascend to the mlf, form a hair-pin bend, turn dorsolaterally, and leave the brain stem dorsal to the spinal tract and nucleus of the trigeminus. The form of neurons in the lateral subnucleus is more diverse. Many of them are the small (about 15 μm) counterpart of neurons in the medial subnucleus, but there are also spheric, oval-shaped and polygonal perikarya of similar sizes. The axonal trajectory is the same as in the medial subnucleus.

There are no direct data as to whether neurons with different forms innervate specific groups of muscles of the jaw joint; however, some indirect inference can be made. The form and distribution of the small version of type 2 neurons within the V–VII nuclear complex are comparable with that described in the frog. This suggests that these neurons supply the intermandibularis by way of the mandibular nerve, and the interhyoideus and the depressor mandibulae by way of the facial nerve. The large trigeminal neurons probably innervate the jaw closing muscles. This is supported by the finding that the adductor mandibulae is supplied by the rostral portion of the ventrolateral trigeminal subnucleus in the *Varanus* (Barbas-Henry and Lohman 1986) and in the pit viper (Moody and Meszler 1980). In this part of the nV the large neurons predominate. We do not have any data about the peripheral target of the type 1 neurons. Their extremely small size suggests that they may innervate intrafusal fibers. As in the frog, jaw closing is controlled by the trigeminus whereas jaw opening is controlled by the facialis.

6.3.3 Bird

In view of the curious nature of the movements of the beak with the kinetic skull and the partial fusion of the nV and nVII, a brief review is inserted here on the innervation of jaw muscles in birds. The description of this chapter relies mainly on the excellent work of Wild and Zeigler (1980) and Berkhoudt et al. (1982) performed on the pigeon, *Columba livia*.

Three muscle groups, classified by their functions, move the avian jaw. These are the protractors, depressor mandibulae and protractor quadrati and pterygoidei, which open the lower and upper jaw, respectively. The retractors, pterygoideus lateralis and pseudotemporalis profundus, and adductors, adductor mandibulae and pseudotemporalis superficialis, close the beak.

These muscles are innervated by the trigeminal-facial nuclear complex (Fig. 8). Wild and Zeigler (1980) divide nV into three subnuclei. The dorsal subnucleus innervates the depressor palpebrae of the lower lid. This muscle forms a sling under the eye bulb and its position and innervation closely resemble the frog's levator bulbi and its motor nucleus. The intermediate subnucleus is the main part of the trigeminus and it innervates the retractors and adductors. Immediately ventral to this main subnucleus, a moderate segregation of neurons forms the ventral subnucleus which supplies the intermandibularis. At the dorsomedial aspect of the main subnucleus a column of motoneurons not completely separated from it innervates the protractors. The beak opening muscles are, therefore, innervated by a common column of neurons. Axons from the rostral part of the column join the trigeminal nerve, whereas axons from its caudal part (the dorsal facial nucleus) leave the brain stem by way of the facial nerve. At the level of the ventral trigeminal nucleus, a separate group of neurons lying more ventrally innervates the suprahyoid muscle group. This is the ventral facial nucleus. The intermandibularis and the suprahyoid muscles are thus supplied by two adjacent nerve groups.

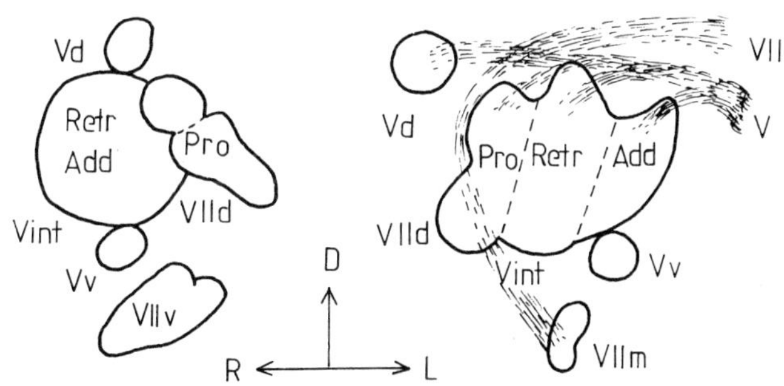

Fig. 8. The combined trigeminal and facial nuclear complex of a bird (*Columba livia*) is shown in sagittal (*left*) and in horizontal (*right*) sections. *Vd*, the dorsal trigeminal subnucleus; *Pro*, *Retr*, *Add*, subnuclei innervating protractor, retractor, and adductor muscles, respectively, in the intermediate trigeminal subnucleus (*Vint*); *VIId*, the dorsal facial subnucleus which merges with the *Pro* section of the intermediate subnucleus of the nV; *Vv* and *VIIv*, the ventral subnucleus of the nV and nVII, respectively; *V* and VII, the trigeminal and facial motor roots. In the middle orientation coordinate ***R*** is the rostral, ***D*** is the dorsal, and ***L*** is the lateral direction. (Modifiedd from Wild and Zeigler 1980 and Berkhoudt et al. 1982)

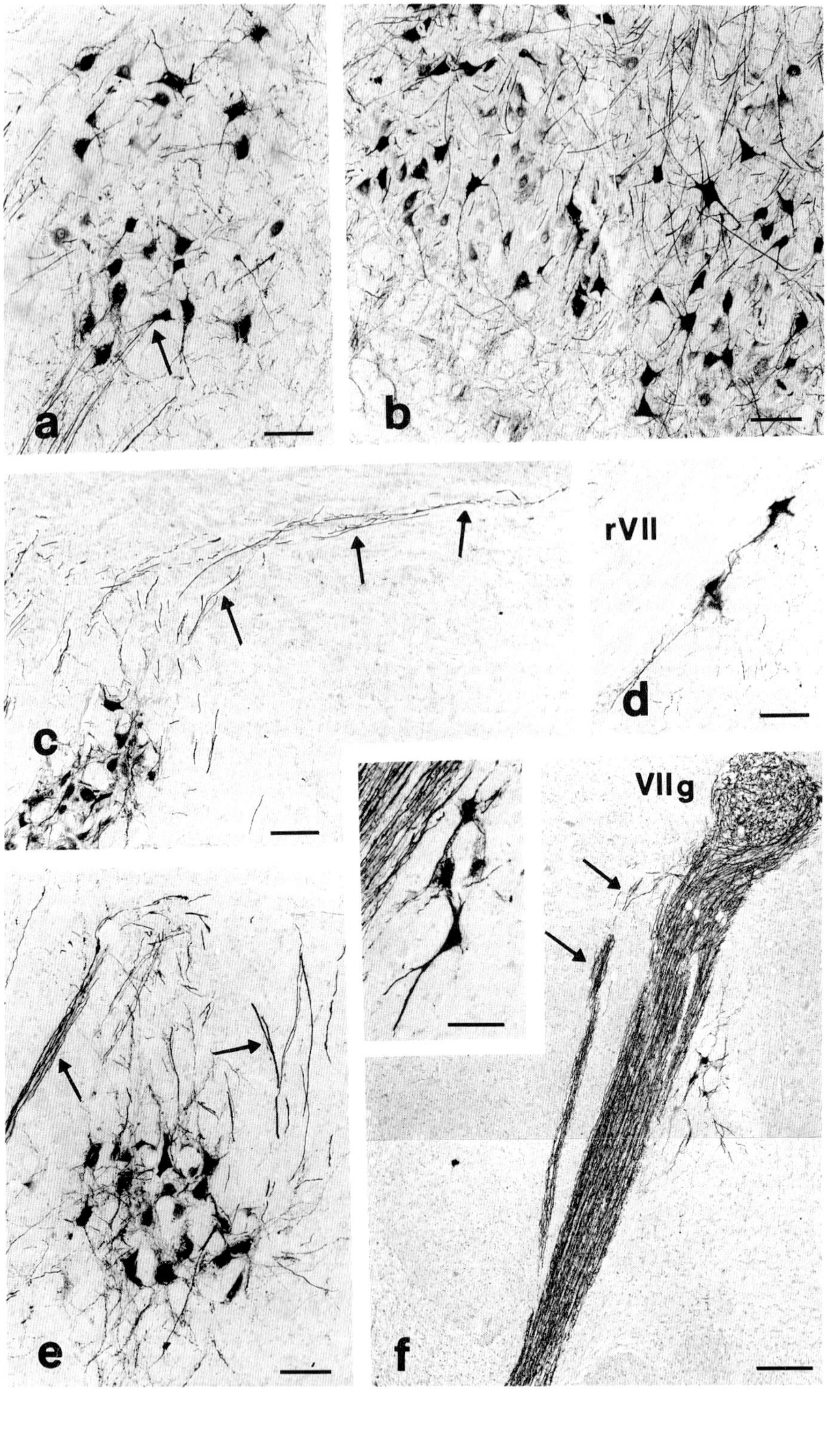
a
b
rVII
c
d
VIIg
e
f

Unfortunately, there are no data about the form, dendritic arborization pattern, and axonal trajectory of this nuclear complex. Some of the HRP specimens of Wild and Zeigler (1980) are suggestive of the presence of dorsal loops formed by the axons as they turn laterally after an initial dorsomedial course. A facial genu, in fact, is shown in the chicken following HRP application to the facial nerve (Ganchrow et al. 1986).

6.4 The Control of Movement at the Secondary Mandibular Joint: The Mammalian Trigeminal Nucleus

Results obtained with recent tracing techniques reveal a close similarity in the organization of the trigeminal nucleus in all mammals investigated (rat: Mizuno et al. 1975; Limwongse and DeSantis 1977; Ibrahim Bin Haji Mohd and Leong 1979; cat: Mizuno et al. 1975; Batini et al. 1976; Landgren and Olson 1976; monkey: Ibrahim Bin Haji Mohd and Leong 1979; Mizuno et al. 1981). Our findings, obtained from rat material with the cobalt technique (Székely and Matesz 1982), are in accordance with these studies and provide data on the morphology of neurons. In the following description we rely mainly on these results.

The trigeminal motor nucleus is an ellipsoid cluster of cells which can be divided into two divisions on a cytoarchitectonical basis. The larger dorsolateral division is the main nucleus (nVm), and the ventromedial is the accessory nucleus (nVa). This latter is also called the retrotrigeminal nucleus, or the α division of the trigeminal nucleus in the old literature (Meeson and Olszewski 1949). It forms the tapering end of the trigeminal nuclear complex.

The neuron population distinctly differs in the two divisions. In the nVm, neurons have polygonal perikarya which measure 45–55 μm in diameter (Fig. 9a, Fig. 10g). The dendrites radiate out in all directions extending beyond the confines of the nucleus. The axon emerges from the ventral aspect of the cell body, follows a straight course to the trigeminal motor root, and continues in the anterior trunk of the mandibular nerve. This type of neuron innervates the four masticatory muscles.

Neurons in the nVa have elongated somata which are oriented in the dorsoventral direction (Fig. 9c,e). A dorsal and a ventral dendritic array emerges from the upper and the lower ends of the perikaryon, but a weak lateral and a medial dendrite group can also be distinguished (Fig. 10e). The dorsal dendrites tend to expand in a fan-like manner whereas the ventral

◁ **Fig. 9a–f.** The trigeminal and facial nuclei of the rat. **a** The main trigeminal nucleus (nVm). Note the ventral origin of axons from perikarya (*arrow*). **b** Photomontage of the main facial nucleus (nVIIm). **c** The rostral part of the accessory trigeminal nucleus (nVa). *Arrows* indicate the hairpin turn of axons. **d** Labeled nVa neurons at the medial aspect of the ascending root of the facial nerve (*rVII*). **e** The middle part of the nVa. *Arrows* indicate the dorsal loop in the axonal trajectory. **f** The ascending root of the facial nerve and nVIIa neurons. Note that the nVIIa axons (*arrows*) do not contribute to the internal genu (*VIIg*) of the facial nerve. In the *inset* the nVIIa neurons are shown with high power. *Calibration bar* is 100 μm in **a–e**; 200 μm in **f**; 50 μm in the inset

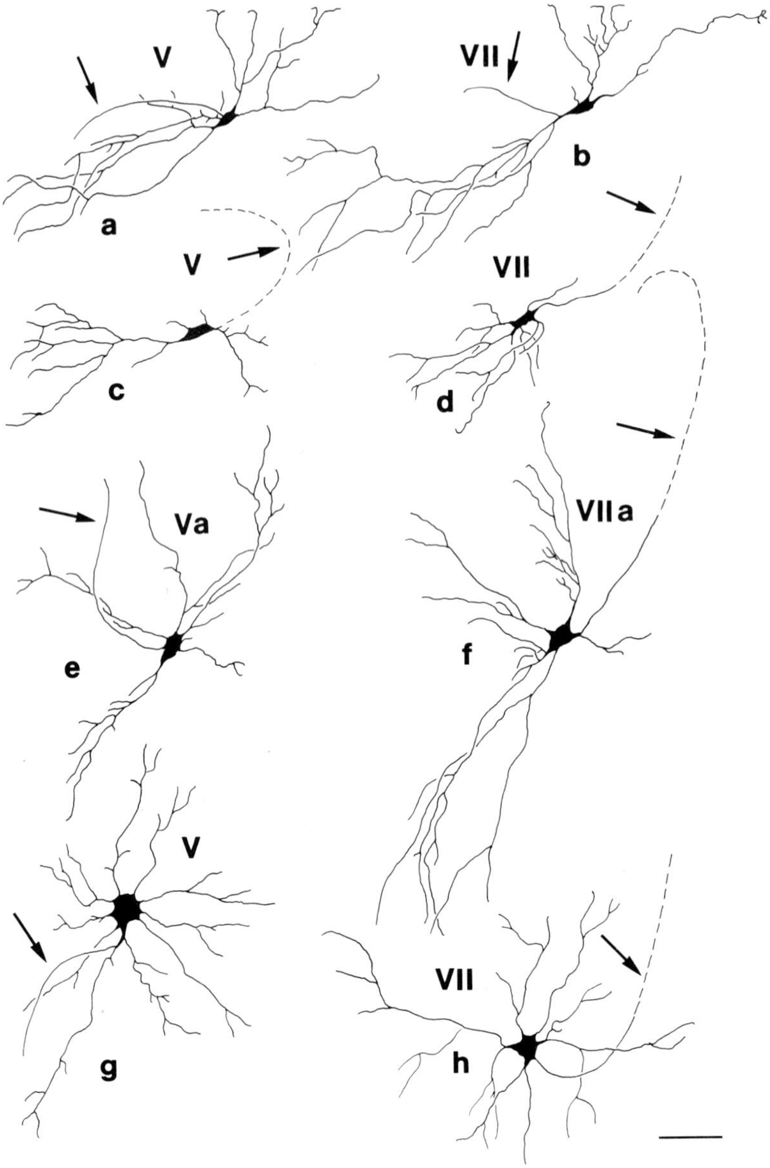

Fig. 10a–h. Camera lucida reconstructions of trigeminal and facial motoneurons. **a**, **b** Frog submaxillaris (**a**) and depressor mandibulae (**b**) neurons. **c**, **d** Lizard, neuron in **c** is from the caudal part of the nV and in **d** from the medial division of the nVII. **e**–**h** Rat. **e**, **f** Neurons from the nVa and VIIa. **g**, **h** Neurons from the nVm and nVIIm, respectively. *Arrows* show the axon. *Calibration bar* is 100 μm

dendrites display the broom-like pattern of arborization. The axons almost always originate in the dorsal part of neurons, follow a dorsally directed curved route, and with a distinct dorsal bend turn ventrally to reach the trigeminal motor root (Fig. 9c). Some of the most medially laying neurons emit their axons toward the midline, they make a hairpin turn at the lateral aspect of the mlf and continue their course in the direction of the motor root (Fig. 9c). Axons of the nVa run in the posterior trunk of the mandibular nerve and innervate the mylohyoid, the anterior digastric, and the transverse mandibular muscles.

Similar morphological differences between motoneurons in the nVm and nVa can be observed in the cat, as shown by Yoshida et al. (1987) with intracellular HRP injections. Although the intracellular labeling reveals more extensive dendritic arbors, the characteristic broom-like arborization pattern of ventral dendrites and the dorsally looping axon can be clearly recognized in their drawing representing a neuron in the nVa. The dorsally looping axons of accessory trigeminal neurons are also shown by Jacquin et al. (1983) in the rat and by Nomura and Mizuno (1983) in the cat.

There is a characteristic somatotopic organization of muscle representation in the trigeminal nucleus which agrees, with little variation, in all of the species listed above. In this organization the temporal muscle is represented dorsally and dorsomedially, the masseter ventrolaterally, and the pterygoid muscles ventromedially in the main nucleus. The mylohyoid muscle representation is in the ventrolateral part of the accessory and the main nucleus, the tensor veli palatini is innervated from the rostral part, and the anterior digastric from the caudal part of the accessory nucleus. The innervating neurons intermingle with the posterior digastric neurons of the accessory facial nucleus.

6.5 The Control of Facial Expression: The Mammalian Facial Nucleus

This nucleus extends from the level of the nVI to the caudal border of the pons, dorsal and caudal to the superior olive (Fig. 12). On the basis of its cytoarchitecture, the main facial nucleus (nVIIm) is divided into five to six subnuclei which innervate the muscles of facial expression in a common topographic organization in a variety of animals investigated (opossum: Dom 1982; mouse: Ashwell 1982; rat: Hinrichsen and Watson 1984; rabbit: Baisden et al. 1987; cat: Kume et al. 1978; monkey: Welt and Abbs 1990). In the general scheme of musculotopic organization, the peioral and nasolabial muscles are represented laterally, the auricular muscles medially, the platysma and anterior neck muscles ventrally, orbital and scalp muscles dorsally. Individual muscles are innervated by longitudinal columns of motoneurons, and each muscle region is represented at all rostrocaudal level within this scheme of organization.

Dorsal and medial to the rostral pole of this nucleus there is a small cluster of neurons which extends rostrally and fuses with the nVa. This cluster is called the dorsal facial nucleus by some investigators and the accessory facial nucleus (nVIIa) by others (Fig. 12). It supplies the stylohyoid and the posterior digastric muscles (Szentágothai 1949; Mizuno et al. 1975).

In our rat material, cobalt labeling of the nVIIm reveals a neuronal morphology which very closely resembles the trigeminal motoneurons in the main nucleus (Fig. 9b). The dendrites radiate out in all directions from a polygonal cell body and the axon usually originates in the ventral part of the soma (Fig. 10h). Almost at their origin, the axons turn dorsally and converge on a point lateral to the main abducens nucleus. Here they form a complicated whirl-like structure as the individual fibers run rostrally along a spiral path (Fig. 9f). This is known as the internal genu of the facial nerve. It is about 1 mm long in the rostrocaudal direction in the rat. The fibers then sharply turn ventrally and constitute the descending root of the facial nerve. Intracellular HRP injections (Shaw and Baker 1985) show similar radially oriented dendritic geometry in the rat and cat facial nucleus. Neurons in the nVIIa are counterparts of neurons in the nVa (Fig. 10f). The axons ascend in the direction of the facial genu and arch back ventrally to join the facial motor root (Fig. 9f).

The nVa and the nVIIa are made up of the same type of neuron and form a common club-shaped structure (Fig. 12). The "head" of the club is formed by the rostral larger part of the accessory trigeminal nucleus, whereas in the "shaft" of the club trigeminal and facial accessory motoneurons intermingle (Fig. 9d). This common nucleus of the trigeminal and facial nerves was first recognized by Szentágothai (1949) and corroborated later by Matsuda et al. (1979). In addition to the rat, it has been found in the guinea pig, cat, dog, and monkey. A facial component of the joint nVa–nVIIa could not be shown in the rabbit in which the posterior belly of the digastric muscle is nonexistent (Matsuda et al. 1979).

6.6 Conclusion

Unlike the relative conservation in the organization of the eye and tongue moving motor nuclei in various vertebrate species, the trigeminal and facial motor nuclei reveal profound changes in phylogenesis. These changes are part of a series of structural transformations involving the orofacial region and are associated with a basic modification of the feeding behavior of the animal (Crompton 1989). One of the salient points of this modification is the capability of mammals for grinding the food, which is a much more complex activity than the simple grasping movement that the amphibian and sauropsidian jaw is capable of performing. Following the distinction made between the two kinds of jaw joints, we suggest a similar distinction and call the anuran and sauropsidian motor centers the primary trigeminal (nV) and facial (nVII) motor nuclei as opposed to the secondary trigeminal and facial nuclei represented by nVm and nVIIm in mammals.

There are a number of changes in the primary trigeminal and facial nuclei as well. Motoneurons in the frog nV, which supply the levator bulbi, are unique not only in their characteristic dendritic geometry but also in the course of their axons in the maxillary and ophthalmic nerves. No other animal species are known in which these nerves carry motor fibers. This type of neuron and the corresponding muscle is absent from the lizard. Nerve and muscle disappear together in phylogenesis; it would be interesting to know if this apparatus can be detected in a vestigial form in reptilian embryos.

On the basis of their disparate dendritic geometry, closer and opener neurons can be distinguished in nV and nVII (see Fig. 10). Opener neurons, which also supply the muscles of the floor of the mouth, whether in the nV or in the nVII, show a remarkable consistency as far as their form and size are concerned in the frog and the lizard. They supply a group of muscles with remarkable similarity not only in form and position but also in function. Closer motoneurons are not as uniform as openers. Although there are mainly size differences, the presence of more than one type of closer neurons suggests that jaw closing is a much more delicate action than opening even at the primary mandibular joint.

These considerations suggest that the control of specific functions of the primary and secondary mandibular joints can be associated with the presence of neurons of characteristic form. Furthermore, neurons with the same, or similar, functions are segregated in common groups. This grouping is especially clear in the case of neurons innervating the levator bulbi and in the innervation of the floor of the mouth and the opener muscles. The grouping of neurons with the same function is beautifully demonstrated by the innervation of the opener muscles of the upper and lower beaks by the trigeminal and facial nerves originating from neurons of the fused trigeminal-facial nucleus.

An interesting feature of neurons in the primary trigeminal and facial nuclei is the dorsally looping axons, or the hairpin turn, in their central trajectory in the lizard. This can be sporadically found also in the frog nV. This curious course of axons can probably be explained by their dorsal origin from the cell body. They take an initial straight course dorsally, or medially, and they have to make a turn in order to leave the brain stem in the lateral direction.

In the secondary trigeminal nucleus, one type of neuron with a dorsally looping axon is strongly reminiscent of the "opener" neurons of the primary trigeminal nucleus. This type constitutes the accessory trigeminal (nVa) and facial (nVIIa) nuclei which form a common column of neurons in mammals. This type of neuron innervates the same kind of muscles as in the frog and the lizard: the floor of the mouth and the opener of the jaw. These muscles are clearly homologous in amphibia, sauropsidia, and mammals (Starck 1982); moreover, they are innervated by the same type of neuron. This coincidence suggests that the type of innervation may be an important cue in deciding the homology between muscle groups of different species.

From this point of view, the disappearance of motoneurons innervating the levator bulbi of the frog also deserves attention. It seems that there is no homologue for this muscle in other species. The musculus orbitalis, which is a smooth muscle and receives sympathetic innervation, is erroneously held to be the homologous derivative of the levator bulbi. As pointed out above, a probable candidate for homology could be the depressor palpebrae inferioris in birds, as far at least as the approximate position of the muscle and the innervating neuron group are concerned. Nevertheless, these two muscles and the corresponding neural apparatus are not found in mammals.

The characteristic "closer" type of neuron of the primary trigeminal nucleus is also lacking from the secondary trigeminal nucleus. They are replaced by the masticatory motoneurons which form the nVm in the mammalian trigeminal nuclear complex. We have referred above to Starck's (1982) notion that a direct homology cannot be found between mammalian and nonmammalian jaw closer muscles. It seems, therefore, to be a feasible suggestion that the amphibian and sauropsidian closer muscles and neurons are replaced by the mammalian masticatory muscles and neurons during phylogenesis. An aspect of the structural evolution of the secondary temporomandibular joint is the appearance of a novel set of muscles, together with a novel motor center, which is capable of performing and controlling the complex masticatory movement.

We do not have sufficient data about the structural and functional complexity of the amphibian and sauropsidian closer muscles to compare them with the mammalian masticatory muscles, which are known to have a very delicate compartmentalization. This has been shown in the pig masseter muscle (Herring et al. 1989) in which motor unit territories are confined to muscle fascicles. The strong localization endows the muscle with the ability to contract its parts differentially according to the continuously changing task presented by the movement between geometrically uneven articular surfaces and the variable consistency of the food. It is known that the appropriate neural command is generated by a central pattern generator (Dubner et al. 1978; Linden 1978; Luschei and Goldberg 1981), and the activity of this generator is modulated by a number of reflexes arising in the muscle and the mucous membrane of the mouth, teeth, and skin of the face (Lund and Olson 1983). Interestingly, these modulatory reflexes are more complicated in the masticatory muscles and are predominantly monosynaptic in nature arising in static and dynamic fusimotor systems. This is in sharp contrast to the jaw opener muscles in which reflexes are primarily generated by mechanoreceptors and are polysynaptically transmitted.

The secondary facial nucleus (nVIIm) and the primary facial nucleus (nVII) have virtually no relation to one another. The form of the neurons and the axonal trajectory are conspicuously different in the two nuclei (Fig. 9f). The nVIIm is the motor center of facial expression. These muscles appear first in mammals during phylogenesis, and it is generally held that they derive from the sphincter colli which differentiates from the superficial sheet of the primordial constrictor muscle. In his comprehensive study (and, to the best of our knowledge, the latest) on the evolution of the facial musculature, Huber (1930) arguing in favor of this view states: "the common innervation through branches of the *N. facialis* remains the only indication that the two muscle groups (superficial and deep) belong together genetically." The novel type of innervation of facial expression muscles takes away "the only indication" from Huber's argument that they would have derived from the superficial sheet of the facial muscle mass. The depressor mandibulae, which differentiates from the deep sheet, is also suggested to contribute to the evolution of the platysma and the stapedius (Starck 1982). But again, the differences in the innervation lead one to seriously question the common origin of the depressor mandibulae and the platysma and, as will be shown in the next chapter, the stapedius has quite a unique nerve supply. On the basis of the type of their innervation it is more probable that the depressor mandibulae is the primordium of the stylohyoideus and posterior digastricus; both are innervated by the nVIIa, whereas the muscles of facial expression and the secondary facial nucleus are novel structures appearing first in mammals.

7 The Muscles of the Middle Ear

Middle ear muscles insert on the auditory ossicles. Nonmammalian tetrapods possess a single auditory ossicle, the columella. It is the derivative of the upper end of the hyoid arch and extends between the skin (tympanic membrane) and the perilymphatic cistern. In sauropsidia, a portion of the depressor mandibulae primordium is detached and forms the extracolumellaris muscle. It is innervated by the facial nerve and stretches the tympanic membrane. In mammals there are two muscles: the tensor tympani muscle innervated by the trigeminal nerve and the stapedius muscle supplied by the facial nerve. They have a very complex function in hearing by acting upon the ossicular chain. The stapedius is regarded as a homologue of the extracolumellaris muscle (Starck 1979).

7.1 The Central Innervation of the Tensor Tympani

In contrast to the classic finding (Borg 1973; Szentágothai 1949) that the tensor tympani motoneurons are localized in the ventral parvicellular portion of the trigeminal motor nucleus, recent tracing techniques applied to a number of animal species (rat and guinea pig: Spangler et al. 1982; rabbit: Takahashi et al. 1984; cat: Mizuno et al. 1982; Friauf and Baker 1985; Shaw and Baker 1983; Keller et al. 1983; monkey: Gannon and Eden 1987) find them outside the traditionally recognized trigeminal motor nucleus. The cells lay ventrolateral to the nucleus stretching in the rostral two thirds of its longitudinal extension. In the rat and the cat, the tensor tympani motoneurons are scattered more widely and extend rostrally up to the level of the inferior colliculus. Some cells appear to intermingle with the trochlearis motoneurons in the cat (Shaw and Baker 1983; Friauf and Baker 1985).

In our rat material, in which the mandibular nerve was labeled with cobalt, we could localize a column of tiny scattered cells, two to five neurons in each section, extending from the caudal level of the inferior colliculus to the caudal one third of the nVm (Fig. 11a). Their position ventral to the trigeminal nucleus and medial to the trigeminal motor root exactly corresponded to the tensor tympani motoneurons described by others in the rat (Spangler et al. 1982). We have, therefore, identified this group of cells with the tensor tympani motoneurons. The mean size of the spindle-shaped or polygonal perikarya is 28–32 μm in the long diameter; that is, they are about half the size of perikarya of the nVm.

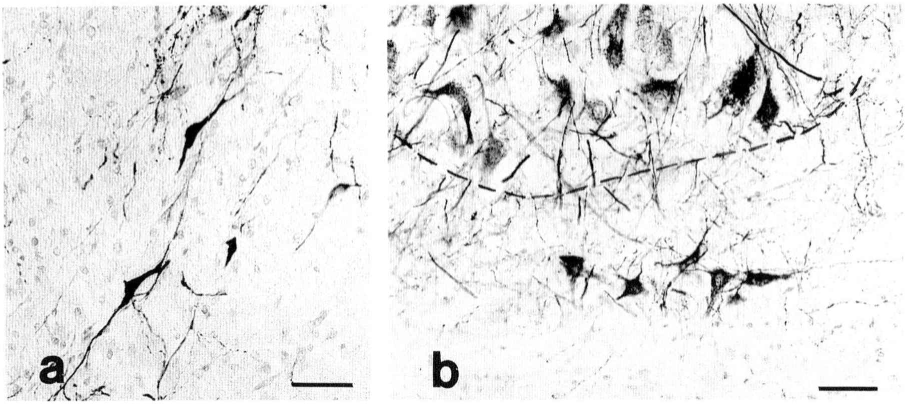

Fig. 11a,b. Neurons of the auditory muscles of the rat. **a** Neurons of the tensor tympani muscle at the level of the trigeminal motor root. **b** Neurons of the stapedius muscle at the ventral aspect (*broken line*) of the nVIIm. *Calibration bar* is 100 μm

A detailed description of the dendritic arborization is given in the beautiful work of Friauf and Baker (1985) in which eight cells injected with HRP are graphically reconstructed and analyzed quantitatively. The dendritic tree extends radially in all directions but none of the dendrite branches penetrate the area of the trigeminal motor nucleus. If a branch encounters the ventral border of the nucleus it immediately changes direction and continues its course horizontally. This observation suggests that the tensor tympani motoneuron pool is distinct from the trigeminal not only in terms of perikaryon size and location, but also the disposition and expansion of the postsynaptic receptive field.

The axon originates from the lateral or dorsal aspect of the soma and with a slight dorsally looping course joins the trigeminal motor root. According to the calculation of Shaw and Baker (1983) somewhat more than 700 motoneurons innervate about 4000 tensor tympani fibers. This results in a very small (1:5.7) innervation ratio. In humans, the fibers of the tensor tympani and tensor veli palatini intermingle. For this reason, these two muscles are considered to be continuous parts of the same muscle mass and they cooperate in the aeration of the tympanic cavity (Lupin 1969). Since the tensor veli palatini is supplied by the nVa (Keller et al. 1983), this relation of the two muscles is rather improbable.

7.2 The Central Innervation of the Stapedius

All recent studies performed with the HRP tracing technique are in agreement that motoneurons innervating the stapedius muscle differ both in location and form from the facial motoneurons in cats (Lyon 1978; Shaw and Baker 1983; Joseph et al. 1985; Guinan et al. 1989; Vacher et al. 1989) and in monkeys (Thompson et al. 1985). According to these findings, the stapedius motoneurons are spread over a number of regions which surround the facial nucleus and the

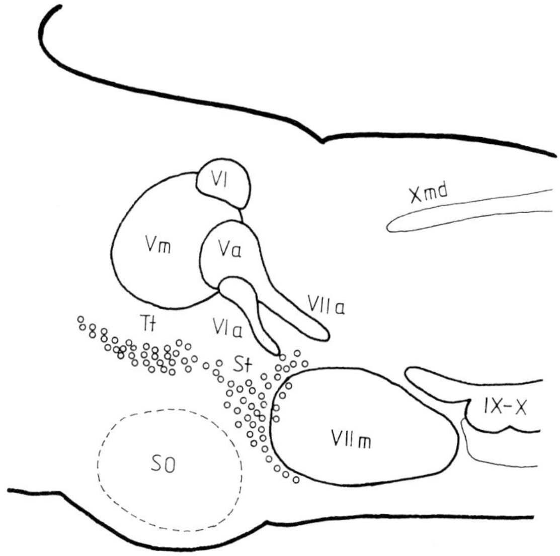

Fig. 12. A medial side view of the topography of motor nuclei in the pons and upper medulla. *Roman numerals* refer to the respective nuclei. *Tt*, the column of the tensor tympani neurons; *St*, the area of the stapedius neurons; *dmX*, the dorsal motor nucleus of the vagus; *SO*, the superior olive

superior olive. Beginning caudally, stapedius neurons first appear ventral to the nVIIm. Their number gradually increases and at the level of the trapezoid body they surround the nVIIm. At the rostral pole of this nucleus, the dorsal and ventral neurons converge and transiently decrease in number to become more numerous again at the descending root of the facial nerve. Here stapedius neurons intermingle with tensor tympani neurons, so that the motoneuron group which innervates the two middle ear muscles constitutes a continuous column (Fig. 12). The middle part of the column is ventral to that part of the nVIIa which innervates the suprahyoid muscles. Cells in the rear end of the column are dispersed and some of them lie in the reticular formation.

Although Vacher et al. (1989) tried to label single neurons through intra-axonal injections, the dendritic arbor did not stain in this experiment. The elongated or polygonal perikaryon is very small, comparable in size with the tensor tympani motoneurons (Fig. 11b). On the basis of the axonal trajectory, Guinan et al. (1989) distinguished a perifacial and an accessory stapedius motoneuron group. Axons of the former neurons travel along the facial nerve axons, whereas axons of the rostrally disposed accessory stapedius neurons follow a dorsally looping course reminiscent of the axonal trajectory seen in the trigeminal and facial accessory neurons. There is an interesting functional distribution which corresponds to this spatial segregation in the sense that neurons which respond to bilateral sound are situated in a narrow band around the nVIIm; those responding to contralateral sound are ventromedial to it, whereas the rostrally laying neurons are sensitive to ipsilateral sound (Vacher et al. 1989).

The number of stapedius motoneurons is surprisingly large. Joseph et al. (1985) report an average of 1163 neurons as counted in three cats. Regarding the number of muscle fibers in the stapedius, which is approximately 1700 (Blevin 1964), this is the smallest motor unit known and suggests a very delicate function of the muscle.

7.3 Conclusion

A well defined middle ear with ossicles and muscles appear first in reptiles. The extracolumellaris muscle derives from a common mass with the depressor mandibulae, but the entirely different functions of the two muscles suggest different sources of innervation. The parvicellular lateral facial nucleus is a likely candidate for the innervation of the reptilian auditory muscle. The mammalian auditory muscles are supplied by a common column of neurons which expands from the caudal part of the mesencephalon to the rostral end of the medulla, ventral and lateral to the nVa and nVIIa (Fig. 12). The form of the perikarya and the trajectory of axons closely resemble that of the trigeminal and facial accessory neurons, but the much smaller size of perikarya distinctly separates the two groups of neurons from one another.

8 Deglutition and Phonation: The Ambiguus Nucleus

The dorsal motor nucleus of the vagus is traditionally included in the efferent nuclear complex of the glossopharyngeal and vagal nerves. Since this nucleus innervates viscera and also possesses a facial component, it will be discussed in the brain stem vegetative system. Here we focus on the central innervation of the branchiogenic striated musculature in the region of the glossopharyngeal and vagal nerves.

8.1 The Innervated Periphery

The glossopharyngeus is the nerve of the third and the vagus of the fourth to sixth branchial arches. The pharynx and the larynx develop from this region and these organs are different in the amphibian-sauropsidian group and in mammals.

The primordial constrictor muscle gives rise to a very complicated set of muscles which are connected to the third to sixth branchial skeleton and pump the water through the gills in fishes (Starck 1982). This muscle group is even more complex in amphibian larvae which perform combined air and water breathing. During the metamorphic climax gill muscles become drastically reduced, a part of them degenerates, and another part fuses with adjacent muscles to form the pharyngeal and the laryngeal musculature (Lubosch 1938).

In the adult frog, four pharyngeal muscles can be recognized (Gaupp 1904). These are the petrohyoideus anterior, which is the only muscle innervated by the glossopharyngeus, and the three petrohyoidei posteriores supplied by the vagus. These muscles, especially the anterior, are powerful pharyngeal constrictors and play a prominent role in deglutition. In addition they take part in inspiration by elevating the larynx and pressing it against the air bubble in the mouth.

The larynx has four muscles: one dilatator and three sphincters. The dilatator opens the laryngeal inlet and the rima glottidis and stretches the vocal cords. The sphincter muscles close the rima glottidis and the laryngeal inlet. The dilatator muscle is innervated by the short (superior) laryngeal nerve and probably receives a few fibers from the long (inferior) laryngeal nerve as well. The sphincters are supplied by the long laryngeal nerve (Gaupp 1904). Since the short laryngeal nerve is the branch of the fourth branchial arch, and the long one belongs to the sixth (the fifth degenerates), the two muscle groups can be regarded as the derivatives of the fourth and sixth arches, respectively (Starck 1982).

A conspicuous change is present in mammals at the region of the glossopharyngeal-vagal nerves. Parallel with the transformation of the primary mandibular joint, the secondary palate and the associated muscles evolve. The separation of the nasal and oral cavities renders possible mastication and passage of air at the same time and suckling. The palatal muscles are innervated partly by the nVa (tensor veli palatini) and partly by the ambiguus nucleus (levator veli palatini). The pharygeal muscles form a muscular tube, and the constrictors can be homologized with the petrohyoideus muscles.

Another evolutionary change appears in the larynx. A large thyroid cartilage differentiates and the arytenoid cartilages become highly movable. The number of laryngeal muscles increases, but their peripheral innervation pattern does not change. The cricothyroid muscle, which can be homologized with the dilatator muscle of the sauropsidian larynx, is innervated by the superior (short) laryngeal nerve and the other laryngeal muscles are supplied by the inferior (long) laryngeal nerve. It is interesting that the fibers of the cricothyroid muscle appear to be the continuation of the caudal constrictor separated only by their line of insertion on the cricoid and thyroid cartilages. Interestingly, the anatomical relation of the dilatator laryngis and the most caudal petropharyngeal muscle is strikingly similar in sauropsidia.

8.2 The Structure and Cytoarchitecture of the Ambiguus Nucleus

8.2.1 Frog

The ambiguus nucleus can be clearly separated into a glossopharyngeal (nIX) and a vagal (nX) component in this animal (Matesz and Székely 1978; Stuesse et al. 1984; Oka et al. 1987a). The nIX forms a small globular aggregation comprising about 40 neurons. This cell aggregate begins at the caudal pole of the main abducens nucleus and extends caudally for a distance of about 300–400 µm. The vagal component of the ambiguus nucleus begins after a short gap of 100–150 µm (Fig. 18a). The caudal pole cannot be easily defined as the ambiguus nucleus and the accessory nerve nucleus overlap in the caudal medulla. If the vagal nerve is soaked with cobalt, the most caudal neuron with a "vagus character" in its form can be found about 300 µm below the obex.

As revealed by the cobalt labeling technique, the shape of the motoneurons very closely resembles that of the facial motoneurons and the type 2 trigeminal motoneurons (Fig. 13a,b and Fig. 17c,e). The perikaryon is oval-shaped or elongated polygonal and varies in size between 20 and 40 µm in the longer diameter. There is a dorsomedial dendritic array with a fan-shaped pattern and a ventrolateral array with the characteristic broom-shaped pattern of arborization. The axon emerges from a ventrolateral dendrite stem, takes an initial dorsal-dorsolateral course, then with a bend turns in the lateral direction toward the root.

The small nIX innervates a single muscle, the petrohyoideus anterior. The three posterior petrohyoidei and the laryngeal muscles receive vagus innervation. The somatotopic organization of the long vagal nucleus was investigated by Stuesse et al. (1984) by applying HRP to a number of peripheral vagus branches, including cardiac, gastric, pulmonary, and laryngeal (longus) nerves. According to their findings, cardiac cells are rostral to pulmonary cells, the gastric branch (probably also esophageal) receives fibers from the entire rostrocaudal extent, whereas laryngeal cells are located more caudally in the nucleus. Since the long laryngeal nerve was labeled, these authors could not obtain data about the representation of the dilatator muscle.

8.2.2 Lizard

There are a number of differences in the organization of the reptilian ambiguus nucleus compared to that of the frog. In our cobalt labeling experiments, labeled glossopharyngeal neurons appear in the caudal continuation of the merged lateral and medial subnuclei of the facial nerve. Since the caudal end of the nVII tends to shift laterally and ventrally, the nIX is the most ventrolaterally positioned branchiomotor nucleus and extends caudally as far as the rostral pole of the nXII (Fig. 18b). The merging of these two nuclei, the facial and glossopharyngeal, has long been recognized in reptiles (Addens 1933). In the early descriptions, the avian nIX is also positioned in such a rostral site and its fusion with the facial nucleus is described in the chicken embryo (Addens 1933).

Labeling of the vagal nerve reveals a sudden break in the organization of the branchiomotor column, as labeled vagal neurons appear lateral and dorsal to the nXII in the obex region (Fig. 18b). A few neurons may lie quite close to the dorsal motor nucleus of the vagus especially in the caudal part of the obex (Fig. 17g), rostrally the separation of the two cell groups is more conspicuous (Fig. 17c). In its caudal end, the nucleus tapers off almost to a single row of nerve cells which can be followed caudal to the level of the commissura infima in the medullospinal junction. Motoneurons innervating the larynx of the gekko (Kennedy 1981a) and *Varanus* (Barbas-Henry and Lohman 1984) are found in a similar dorsal position at the level of the hypoglossal neurons. The latter study describes a few vagal neurons rostral to the nXII. They occupy a more ventral position and are interpreted as preganglionic neurons. Very probably, these neurons represent the "scattered neurons" that we describe later and do not belong to the branchiomotor column. Data available from reptilian material suggest considerable species differences, but the wide separation of the nIX and nX seems to be a common feature in the reptilian brain.

Concerning neuronal morphology, the labeling of glossopharyngeal neurons was not sufficiently complete for a detailed description of the dendritic arbor. Nevertheless the shape and size of the perikaryon are comparable to those of the facial motoneuron in the medial subnucleus and of the type 2 motoneurons in the trigeminal nucleus (Fig. 13c). The cell body is oval or elongated polygonal and the axon arises from the dorsal aspect of the neuron.

The axonal trajectory is the same as in the facial nerve: the axons run in the dorsomedial direction, make a hairpin turn at the lateral side of the mlf, and course toward the lateral side of the medulla. Fibers from the rostral part of the nucleus do not emerge from the brain stem at the level of rootlet

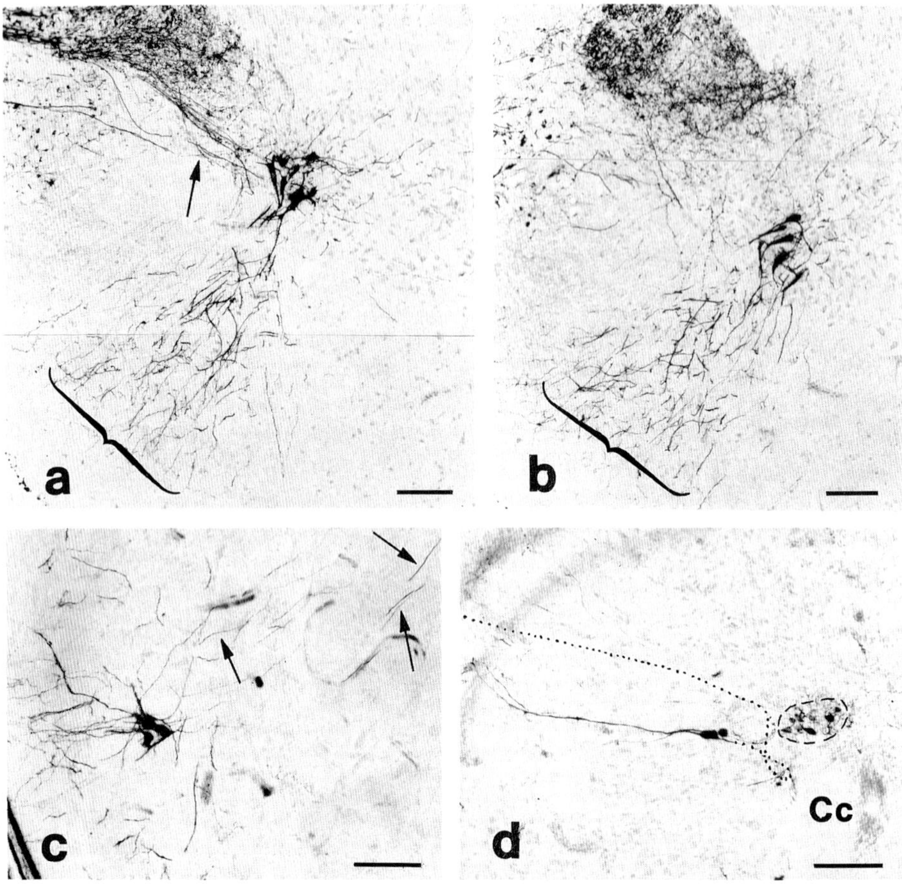

Fig. 13a–d. The glossopharyngeal and the vagal nuclei of the frog and lizard. **a**, **b** Frog (photomontages). In **a** the nIX, in **b** the nX is shown. *Brackets* indicate the broom-like ventrolateral dendrites; *arrows* in **a** point at the axons. **c**, **d** Lizard. In **c** the nIX is shown; *arrows* point at axons which ascend in the direction of the medial longitudinal fasciculus. In **d** a vagus neuron is shown, the *dotted line* indicates the course of the axon. *Cc*, the central canal; the dorsal motor nucleus of the vagus is demarkated by *broken line*. Calibration bar is 100 μm

formation but turn and run caudally underneath the pia mater and form a common root with more caudal fibers.

Neurons in the nX are smaller, approximately 19 μm in the long diameter, and the body is more elongated than in nIX (Fig. 13d; Fig. 17f). The dendritic arbor is bipolar and lies in the horizontal plane presenting a medial and lateral dendritic array in the obex region. The medial dendrites point in the direction of the caudal narrow part of the fourth ventricle, the lateral dendrites extend to the surface in a broom-like arborization pattern. The axons emerge from the medial aspect of neurons and, due to the dorsal position of the nucleus, turn ventrally in the direction of the mlf. Here, with a hairpin loop, they turn back dorsally, pass by the dorsal motor nucleus of the vagus, and with a lateral bend run toward the root exit.

According to our observations made on the sand lizard in cobalt labeling experiments, the glossopharyngeal and vagal nuclei differ from one another not only in their relative positions in the brain stem but also in their cellular composition. Although the general form of neurons in the two nuclei is very similar, vagal neurons are conspicuously smaller than glossopharyngeal neurons. The question is whether the two nuclei can be regarded as a single ambiguus nucleus according to the classic definition?

Unfortunately, a detailed study on the somatotopic organization of the glossopharyngeal-vagal nuclear complex of reptiles, which would be of help in deciding how this nuclear complex is comparable to the mammalian ambiguus nucleus, is not available, and contradictory descriptions in the early literature add to the confusion rather than help disentangle the question. In recent descriptions, the position of laryngeal motoneurons in the gekko (Kennedy 1981a) exactly corresponds to the site where we localize vagus motoneurons in the sand lizard, but this author does not pronounce a view about the gekko's glossopharyngeal-vagal ambiguus nucleus. In *Varanus*, Barbas-Henry and Lohman (1984) distinguish three cell groups in the upper medulla: The first is a large-celled glossopharyngeal component which topographically corresponds to the nIX in our experiment. The second is a rostral vagal component which consists of preganglionic neurons and is continuous with the alleged inferior salivatory nucleus. These cells represent the "vegetative scattered neurons" described in Chap. 10. Third, is a second vagal component dorsal and caudal to the large-celled glossopharyngeal component, corresponding to the rostral pole of the separate nX in our experiment. Therefore, neither Barbas-Henry and Lohman's (1984) *Varanus* material nor our findings in the sand lizard make possible the distinction of the ambiguus nucleus in the conventional sense.

8.2.3 Rat

Although the mammalian nucleus ambiguus has been recognized and its position correctly described in early works (van Gehuchten 1898b; Ramon y Cajal 1909), there is still much misconception concerning the relation of this nucleus to other brain stem nuclei even with the application of recent tracing techniques. The ambiguus nucleus is often regarded as the direct continuation of the nVII in the rabbit (Lawn 1966a,b) and the bat (Schwitzer et al. 1981), and this rostral part is denoted as the nucleus retrofacialis innervating pharynx and larynx muscles in the cat (Gacek, 9975; Kalia and Mesulam 1980b; Yoshida et al. 1981) and in the rat (Kalia and Sullivan 1982). In its caudal part the ambiguus nucleus is brought in direct relation with the accessory nerve nucleus in sheep, horse, and cattle using the retrograde degeneration technique (Flieger 1964, 66, 67), and the presence of accessorius fibers in the cervical vagal nerve is indicated in HRP tracing experiments in the cat (Kalia and Mesulam 1980a) and the rat (Kalia and Sullivan 1982). In these studies vagal motoneurons were localized in the ill-defined retroambigualis nucleus (Olszewski and Baxter 1954) and in the dorsomedial nucleus of the spinal cord. These contradictions stem primarily from the lack of an exact definition of the

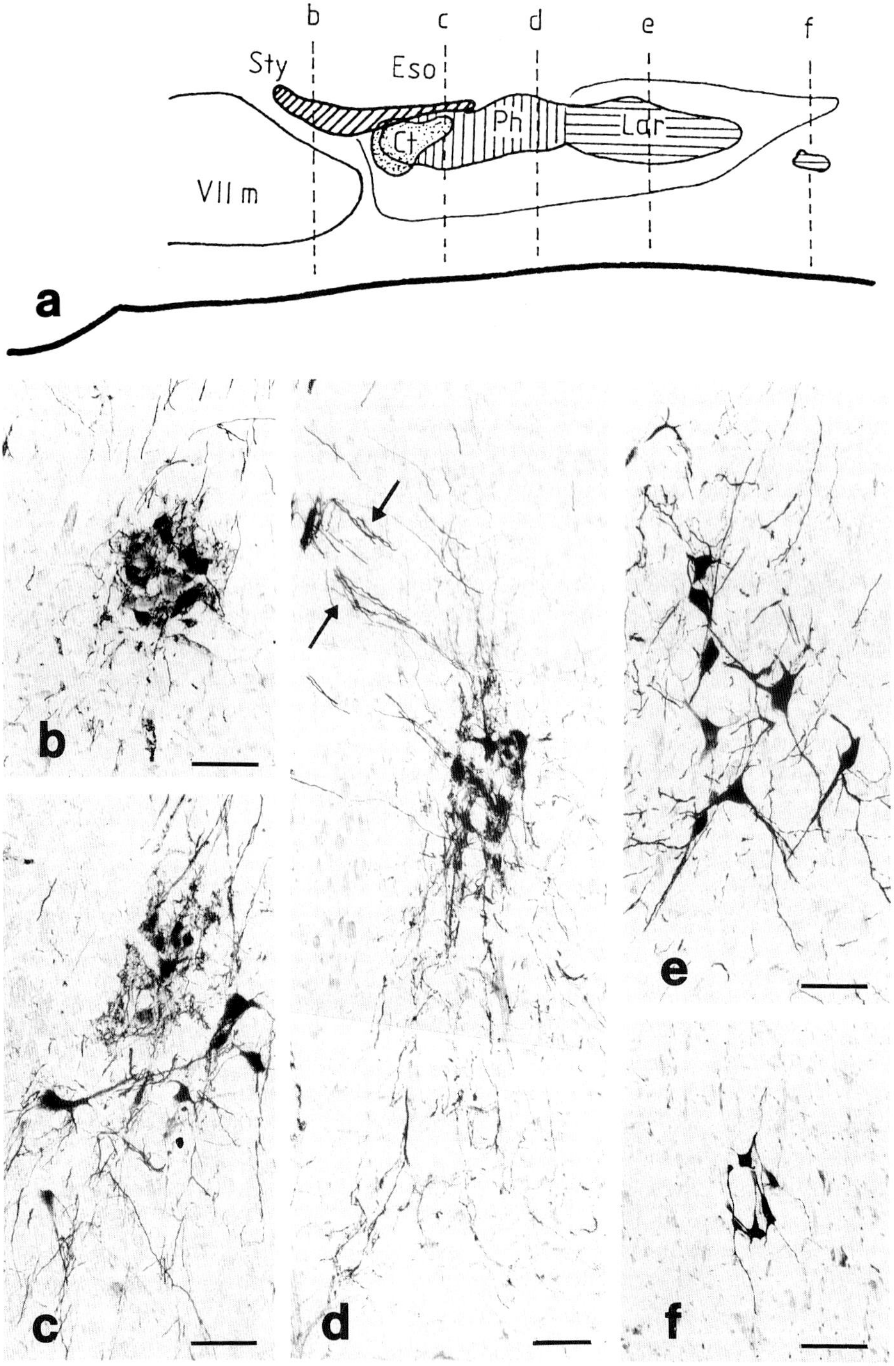

Fig. 14a–f. The ambiguus nucleus of the rat. **a** Extent of the ambiguus nucleus. The compact formation is *thickly hatched*, the semicompact formation is *vertically hatched*, and the loose formation is *horizontally hatched*. Muscle representations are indicated by *letters*; the data are taken from Bieger and Hopkins (1987). *Sty*, stylopharyngeus; *Eso*, striated muscles of the esophagus; *Ct*, cricothyroideus (*stippled*); *Ph*, constrictor pharyngis; *Lar*, laryngeal muscles.

topography of the ambiguus nucleus and the insufficient morphological criteria of glossopharyngeal and vagal motoneurons.

From a beautiful series of HRP labeling experiments performed on rats, pigs, and monkeys, Hopkins and colleagues (Hopkins et al. 1984; Gwyn et al. 1985; Bieger and Hopkins 1987; Hopkins 1987) provide what seems to be the best description of the position, cytoarchitecture, and organization of the ambiguus nucleus. Our own data, obtained from cobalt experiments on rats, closely correspond to this description and supplement it with observations on the morphology of constituent neurons and on the topographical relation of the nucleus ambiguus to other cranial nerve nuclei. The present description relies mainly on these data.

8.2.3.1 The Position and Structure of the Ambiguus Nucleus

The ambiguus nucleus, as we intend to define it, begins at the level of the caudal one third of the nVIIm and terminates in the medullospinal junction at the rostral level of the pyramidal decussation (Fig. 14a; Fig. 18c). This extent encompasses a distance of about 2500 μm in our material of young rats. There is a large variety of distances given in the literature in different, but even in the same, species. Since distance measurements in histological preparations are dependent on a number of variables, we rather refer to adjacent structures than distances when defining the sites of various parts of the ambiguus nucleus.

The structural heterogeneity of the ambiguus nucleus was already recognized in early works and four subdivisions were distinguished (van Gehuchten 1898b; Marinesco and Parhon 1917; Molhant 1912; Lawn 1966a,b). They are unambiguously defined by Bieger and Hopkins' (1987) HRP labeling experiments and by our cobalt tracing material (Matesz and Szekely 1983). The rostralmost division is the compact formation which is composed of relatively small, 25–30 μm, tightly packed neurons dorsal to the nVIIm (Fig. 14b). The aggregation of neurons occupies a roundish slightly oval area with a diameter of about 200 μm at its largest point. The dendritic arbor is mainly confined to this area and the majority of dendrites are seen in cross-section in our horizontally cut specimens, indicating longitudinal extension of dendrite branches. This, in fact, is demonstrated in Beiger and Hopkins' (1987) report on histological specimens cut in the sagittal plane.

Slightly behind the caudal pole of the nVIIm, a few larger (35–40 μm) cells appear ventral to the compact formation. These neurons present polygonal slightly elongated somata from which the dendrites emanate mainly in the ventral and dorsal directions (Fig. 14c). The number of large cells gradually

◁ **Fig. 14** (*continued*). The *thin line* demarcates the external formation. *Broken lines* indicate the level of the subjacent photographs labeled with identical letters. **b** The rostral part of the compact formation. **c** A few large neurons represent the semiloose formation under the compact formation. **d** The caudal part of the semiloose formation (photomontage). Note the dorsoventral orientation of dendrites and the loop formation by the initially ascending axons (*arrows*). **e** Neurons in the loose formation. **f** Small neurons in the caudal pole of the ambiguus nucleus. *Calibration bar* is 100 μm increases and they intermingle with small cells, and the compact formation goes over without sharp boundaries into the semicompact formation. The cross-sectional extent of the nucleus also enlarges and a very definite dendritic field can be observed oriented in the dorsoventral direction. At the rostral pole of the nXII, the large cells predominate, and the ventral dendrites reach the surface in a broom-like arrangement of dendritic bundles (Fig. 14d).

In the obex region where the fourth ventricle begins to close and form the central canal, the large polygonal and ovoid cells are dispersed and after a few cell-free sections they reappear in clusters (Fig. 14e). Two to three such clusters are formed in the closed part of the medulla, and at the level of the commissura infima small cells are found again intermingled with large cells. This caudal part is called the loose formation of the ambiguus nucleus. Approaching the caudal pole of the nXII, the number of neurons rapidly decreases and first the large then the small cells disappear. After a gap of about 150 μm, the small cells reappear and, in a single strand, they can be followed as far as the rostral level of the pyramidal decussation (Fig. 14f). This caudal tail of the nucleus contains no more than 10–12 neurons. An external formation of the ambiguus nucleus is also distinguished in the literature. Since it presumably contains preganglionic neurons we shall deal with it later.

The axonal trajectory is very characteristic in all parts of the nucleus and closely resembles that seen in the nVa and nVIIa. As a rule, the axon arises from the dorsal aspect of the neuron and runs in the direction of the mlf. Anywhere between the nucleus and the mlf, the axons sharply turn ventrolaterally and join one of the several fascicles formed by the axons of ambiguus neurons.

8.2.3.2 Somatotopic Organization of the Ambiguus Nucleus

There have been many debates in the literature as to the question of the representation of visceral and muscular innervation in the ambiguus nucleus. According to the present state of conflicting opinions, visceral innervation to the heart arises from the so-called external formation. Since we did not investigate this question, the present description of the innervation of striated muscles relies mainly on the work of Bieger and Hopkins (1987) made on the rat. As the rat misses certain palatal (levator veli palatini and palatoglossus) and pharyngeal (superior constrictor) muscles, some species differences can be expected if a similarly detailed study is performed on different mammals.

As indicated in Fig. 14a, the rostralmost part of the ambiguus nucleus, which consists of small neurons, innervates the stylopharyngeus muscle. This approximately corresponds to what is found in the cat for the same muscle (van Loveren et al. 1985), and these neurons are coexistent with neurons of the cat levator veli palatini (van Loveren et al. 1983). The representation of striated muscles of the esophagus continues caudally in the dorsal part of the compact formation comprising small neurons. A rostrocaudal sequence in the arrangement of neurons is not evident following injections of HRP into the cervical, thoracic, and subdiaphragmatic sections of the esophagus. However, only a crude rostrocaudal organization is revealed by the cervical esophagomotor neurons which are predominantly localized in a cowl-like envelope around the rostral part of the compact formation. As for the most part similar representation of the esophageal musculature is described for the dog (Hudson and Cummings 1985).

Coexistent with the esophagus is the representation of the pharynx but ventral to the esophagomotor neurons in the field of larger cells. Within the pharyngeal field in its most rostral portion, the cricothyroid muscle is represented. The dissociation of the area of representation of this muscle from the rest of the larynx muscles is first described by Szentágothai (1943) in the cat, and confirmed by many authors in a variety of animals. Szentágothai interprets the rostral representation of the cricothyroid muscle by its having detached from the lower constrictor pharyngis muscle. This view is advocated also by Schweizer et al. (1981) working on bats. Interestingly, the localization of thyropharyngeal motoneurons is coexistent with the cricothyroid muscle representation, whereas the hypopharyngeal (middle constrictor) muscle is represented all over the semicompact formation.

The innervation of the intrinsic laryngeal muscles originates in the loose formation. A rostrocaudal myotopical arrangement can be shown in the representation of these muscles (Szentágothai 1943; Okubo et al. 1987). In the loose formation, therefore, the most rostrally represented muscle is the posterior cricoarytenoideus, followed by the thyroarytenoideus, the lateral cricoarytenoideus, and the interarytenoideus as the most caudally represented muscle.

Disregarding a few minor details, the old statement that the ambiguus nucleus consists of three subdivisions: the esophagomotor compact formation, the pharyngomotor semicompact formation, and the laryngomotor loose formation, is roughly correct as far as the innervation of striated muscles is concerned.

8.3 Conclusion

The ambiguus nucleus is the most frequently studied and the most variously described structure of all cranial nerve nuclei. Concerning its structure and function, it is not a unanimously segregated group of neurons as are the other motor nuclei. The nucleus actually owes its name to the ill-defined borders in the ventrolateral reticular formation of the medulla (Krause 1876; cited by Bieger and Hopkins 1987). The large variability of its position and structure in different species, and in the opinion of different authors, makes it an ambiguous nucleus indeed. In order to try to resolve the many ambiguities that still persist, we take into account the common features found in the different species investigated. In this effort we want to consider only the innervation of striated muscles and the morphology of the related ambiguus motoneurons.

8.3.1 Species Differences

The glossopharyngeal-vagal complex innervates muscle groups which are involved in deglutition and (in mammals) phonation. It is clear that these functions greatly vary in different species. Deglutition is performed by quite different muscle mechanisms in animals without a palate compared to animals in which the oral and nasal cavities are separated and the capability of mastication is developed. These organs and muscles are the derivatives of the third to sixth branchial arches which develop in very different ways in species adapted to different habitats.

One would expect the simplest structure of the IX–X nuclear complex in fishes without laryngeal phonation were it not for the delicate control of the gill apparatus. Probably because of difficulties involved in labeling peripheral nerves with tracer dyes, there are few reports on the structure of cranial nerve nuclei in these animals. It is known that the skate has a long dorsomedial motor column which emits efferent fibers to the VII, IX, and X nerves, but the glossopharyngeal component is missing from the ventrolateral motor nucleus which innervates branchiogen muscles and can be homologized with the ambiguus nucleus (Barry 1987). In the goldfish (Morita and Finger 1987), the glossopharyngeal-vagal complex contains a median, a paramedian, and a lateral motor column. The median column innervates primordial subdiaphragmatic viscera, the paramedian column consists of loosely scattered neurons of the heart, and the lateral column innervates pharyngeal muscles and the chewing organ. The relatively diffuse localization of cardiac neurons outside the dorsomedial motor column is an interesting feature in its resemblance to innervation of the mammalian heart (see Hopkins 1987).

In plethodontine salamanders the situation is made much more complicated by the projectile tongue, which plays a key role in apprehension of prey. The posterior subnucleus of the extremely elongated nVII, which innervates the complex interhyoideus muscle group, overlaps the nIX and the rostral part of the nX, and morphologically similar neurons of these nuclei are intermingled (Roth and Wake 1985). The glossopharyngeal-vagal neurons innervate the subarcualis rectus muscle which is a powerful tongue protractor. In these animals, the nVII, nIX and nX form a common nuclear complex.

The frog presents the first separated dorsal (ndmX) and ventrolateral (nIX and nX) motor nuclei, although many small efferent neurons are intermingled with larger ones in the ventrolateral nucleus. The nIX and nX are entirely separated: a small spherical group of neurons (nIX) innervates the petrohyoideus anterior. This muscle is also separated from the more caudal pharyngeal and laryngeal muscles which are innervated by the relatively long column of vagal neurons.

The nVII and nIX are fused in the lizard (Ariëns Kappers et al. 1936; Schwab 1979; Barbas-Henry and Lohman 1984; Székely and Matesz 1988). The facial nucleus contributes to the innervation of the depressor mandibulae, the interhyoideus, and the dilatator tubae, and these structures are also the main innervation area of glossopharyngeal motor fibers (Gillapsy 1954; Soliman 1964; Starck 1982). Another curiosity is the complete dissociation of the nIX and nX in the lizard (Székely and Matesz 1988). Whereas the nIX is found in its classic position in the ventrolateral nuclear column, the nX is relatively small and is separated from this column in its position dorsal to the nXII and lateral to the dorsal motor nucleus of the vagus. The "specific visceral" component of the vagus is also small and is in a similar position in *Varanus*

(Barbas-Henry and Lohman 1984) and in the gekko (Kennedy 1981a). The relatively small nX correlates with the greatly reduced pharyngeal musculature of reptiles (Lubosch 1938), which compels the animal to raise its head for the assistance of gravity in the act of swallowing. The nIX, therefore, has no topographical relation to nX.

In mammals the two nuclei, nIX and nX, extensively overlap, their neurons intermingle in a large part of the nucleus ambiguus. There is, however, disagreement as to the extent of the nucleus, and considerable ambiguity results from the undiscriminating adoption of two names: the nucleus retrofacialis and the nucleus retroambigualis. The first name may have derived from the failure to recognize the most rostral part of the ambiguus nucleus overlying the facial nucleus in nuclear stained specimens and, as one can infer from Taber's (1961) description, the retrofacial nucleus probably corresponds to the rostral semicompact part of the ambiguus nucleus. The use of this name, especially in the form of "ambiguus-retrofacial complex" unnecessarily increases the number of terms and adds to the confusion. The nucleus retroambigualis is even more ill-defined and inconsistently used in modern literature. There is no claim for its contribution to the vagus nerve in early descriptions in which the nucleus is regarded as the medullary homologue of the spinal intermediolateral cell column (Olszewski and Baxter 1954; Taber 1961). According to Kalia and Mesulam (1980a,b) the nucleus retroambigualis is found lateral to the ambiguus nucleus, and its caudal part which extends into the spinal cord contributes to the vagal nerve. This claim was not corroborated. Bieger and Hopkins (1987) also questioned the validity of using the names retrofacial and retroambigual nuclei.

8.3.2 Cytoarchitecture of the Ambiguus Nucleus

The glossopharyngeal-vagal nuclear complex consists of the same type of neuron that is found in the nVII and the second type of neuron of the nV in the frog. That is, a fan-like dorsomedial, a broom-like ventrolateral dendritic array, and a hair-pin bend in the initial dorsolateral course of the axon characterize the morphology of neurons. Similar neuronal morphology is recorded in the dissociated glossopharyngeal and vagal nuclei of the lizard, and a pronounced hairpin loop is invariably present in the course of axons. It is interesting to note that a similar loop is seen in the course of axons in the facial and glossopharyngeal nuclei in salamanders (Roth et al. 1988).

In the rat, the ambiguus nucleus is not the direct continuation of the nVIIm, as generally described, but rather it is in a common rostrocaudal line, with an intervening gap, with the nVa and nVIIa (Figs. 12, 18c). On the basis of its position, one may expect to find ambiguus neurons that are morphologically similar to accessory trigeminal and facial neurons. Concerning the axonal trajectory the initial dorsomedial course and the hairpin loop are invariably presented by all ambiguus neurons, but the dendritic pattern which is comparable to the accessory trigeminal and facial neurons is shown only by the cells in the semicompact formation of the nucleus. There are also a number of polygonal neurons with radially oriented dendrites and middle-sized neurons with rostrocaudal dendrite orientations in the compact formation. Unfortunately, there are no sufficient data to correlate the functional organization and the neuronal morphology in the ambiguus nucleus, but we may make some inference on the basis of Hopkins (1987) and our (Matesz and Székely 1983) observations made in the rat. Neurons which strongly resemble the accessory trigeminal and facial neurons belong very probably to the pharyngeal constrictors. This type of neuron is found in the semicompact formation and this is the site where the pharyngeal constrictors are represented. As the shape and arrangement suggest, the pharyngeal constrictors derive from the caudal part of the primordial constrictor muscle. In their origin these muscles show a kinship with the suprahyoid muscles which derive also from the same muscle mass. These muscles are functionally closely related and are innervated by a common type of neuron.

The middle-sized neurons with rostrocaudal dendrite orientation in the compact formation innervate the stylopharyngeal, palatal, and esophageal muscles. These muscles suspend the pharynx and shorten when they contract. The work of van Loveren et al. (1983) suggests that the levator of the soft palate receives innervation from this neuron group. The caudal part of the compact formation supplies the striated muscle coat of the esophagus. We have no data about the origin of these muscles; we can only state that they receive innervation from a common type of neuron which forms a continuous column. Nevertheless an aside may be made: these muscles are mainly longitudinally oriented and they shorten the upper segment of the alimentary canal and play a prominent part in the act of deglutiation. The palatal muscles and the striated esophageal muscles are absent from amphibia and sauropsidia (Lubosch 1938). These muscles, the middle sized neurons, and the compact formation of the ambiguus nucleus also cannot be found in these animals.

Finally, the intrinsic muscles of the larynx are innervated by the caudal part of the ambiguus nucleus. (The cricothyroid muscle is probably not a true larynx muscle but a part of the caudal pharyngeal constrictor and receives the nerve supply from the semicompact area of the ambiguus nucleus.) The large polygonal neurons are found in greatest number in this part of the nucleus. According to the present state of our knowledge, the loose formation innervates only the muscles of the larynx. These muscles are poorly developed in nonmammalian tetrapods and this may be the reason that the presence of large polygonal neurons is not conspicuous in their vagal nucleus.

We postpone the consideration of the external formation and the small neurons of the ambiguus nucleus to a later chapter.

8.3.3 The Relation to the Accessory Nerve Nucleus

There is a large body of widely contradictory data in the literature on how the ambiguus nucleus also contains an accessory nerve component. In our cobalt material, we could make a clear distinction between vagal and accessory nerve motoneurons on a neuromorphological basis in all three species investigated. We want to emphasize here and show in detail in the next chapter that there is no relation whatsoever between the nuclei of these two cranial nerves.

Considering only the innervation of striated muscles, the following picture emerges concerning the organization of the glossopharyngeal-vagal nuclear complex. There is a large-celled part which is the continuation of the trigeminal and facial nuclei in submammalian tetrapods. This corresponds to the semi-loose and loose components in mammals. With their elongated perikarya and dorsoventral dendritic orientation, many of these neurons are counterparts of the trigeminal and facial neurons in amphibia and reptiles, and of the accessory trigeminal and facial neurons in mammals. Reptiles possess a rudimentary vagal component probably because of their poorly developed caudal pharynx. The compact component is added to the glossopharyngeal-vagal complex in mammals. This component innervates novel structures: longitudinally oriented palatal and esophageal muscles in the oral part of the alimentary canal. These interspecies differences will be further discussed in the last chapter.

9 The Control of Head Movements: The Accessory Nerve Nucleus

9.1 The Periphery

Fishes do not move their heads, and in animals with a real neck the spinal nerves also contribute to the control of head movements. With this title, however, we want to emphasize the functional change that occurred in the accessory nerve area during phylogenesis. The classification of this nerve, its nucleus of origin, and the innervated muscle group is no less ambiguous than the glossopharyngeal-vagal complex. The developmental history of the accessory nerve and its muscles is excellently summarized by Krammer et al. (1987).

The first trace of a muscle comparable with the "trapezius group" of higher order animals is found in telostean fishes (Lubosch 1938; Starck 1982). It can be deduced from the dorsal part of the primordial constrictor superficialis muscle which is innervated by the glossopharyngeal and vagal nerves. A group becomes segregated and extends ventrally from the dorsal fascia to the branchial arches: the levatores arcuum branchialium muscles. The most caudal bundles of this group insert on the shoulder girdle and are innervated by a branch of the vagus, hence the name accessory nerve (to the vagus). A comparable muscle present in amphibia is the capiticlavicularis, or cucullaris. It arises from the occipital synchondrosis, inserts on the scapula, and is innervated by a branch of the vagus: the accessory nerve.

Sauropsidia present a real neck and the insertion of these muscles shifts ventrally to the thorax and to the secondary sternum. Two muscles of the trapezius group differentiate: the capiticleidoepisternalis and the capitidorso-clavicularis. This latter muscle receives spinal nerves but there is an independent accessory nerve for the innervation of the former muscle.

The general mammalian situation is represented by the familiar trapezius and sternocleidomastoideus muscles; each of them can be variously subdivided in different species. A well defined accessory nerve innervates these muscles; the trapezius receives also spinal nerves as it expands over the dorsum.

On the basis of these comparative anatomical data, muscles of the so called trapezius group are regarded as "specific visceral" muscles, the accessory nerve and its nucleus "specific visceromotor" nerve and nucleus which are parts of the glossopharyngeal-vagal complex. In accordance with this view, the several existing investigations in this field conclude with a variety of suggestions on how the accessory nerve nucleus (nXI) is the direct continuation of the ndmX (Flieger 1967), of the ambiguus nucleus (Holomanova et al. 1972; Romanes 1940), and of the hypoglossal nucleus (Flieger 1967). Kalia and Mesulam

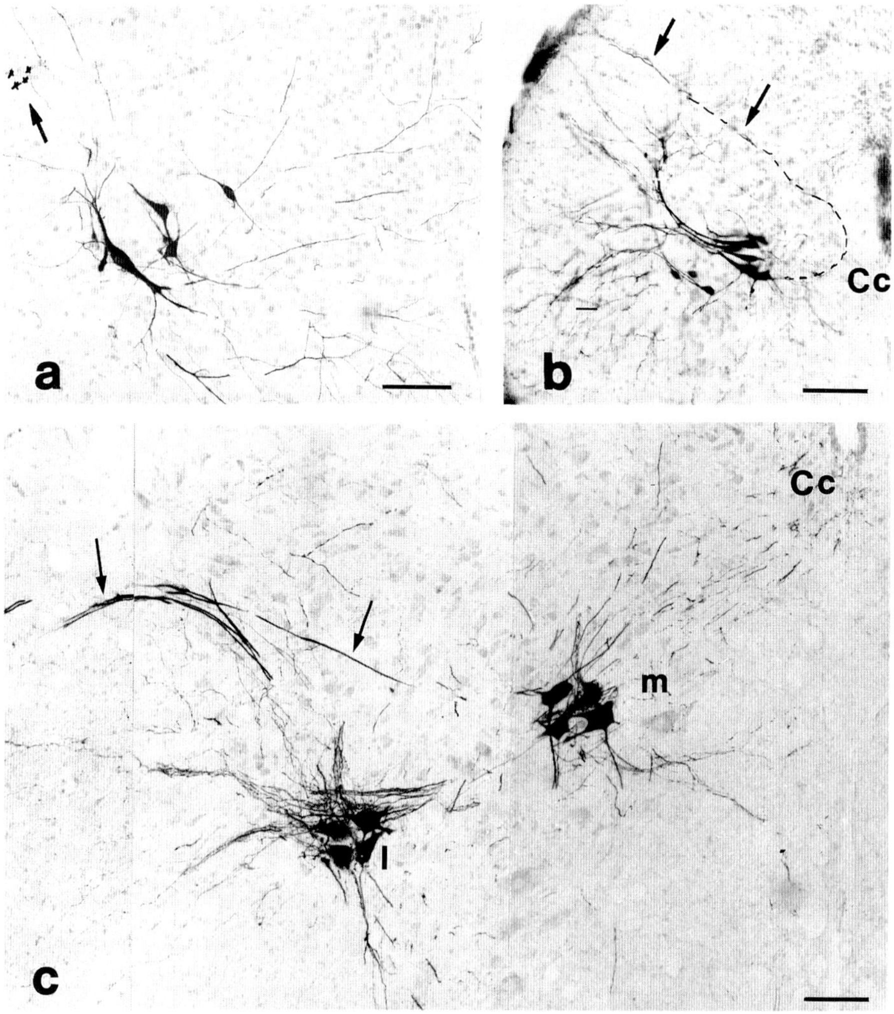

Fig. 15a–c. The accessory nerve nucleus. **a** Frog; *arrow* points at a few cross-sections of ascending axons (retouched). **b** Lizard; *arrows* and *broken line* indicate the axonal trajectory. **c** Rat; the medial (*m*) and the lateral. (*l*) columns of the accessory motoneurons are shown; *arrows* point at the axons. *Co*, central canal. *Calibration bar* is 100 μm

(1980a) assumed the presence of a spinal ambiguus nucleus in order to find a structure for the (vagal) accessory nerve motoneurons. According to the current view, the accessory nerve nucleus has a medullary (ambiguus nucleus) component and a spinal component. On the basis of neuronal morphology we investigate these controversies below.

9.2 The Accessory Nerve

In amphibia, the glossopharyngeal, vagal, and accessory nerves emerge with three to four readily identifiable distinct roots which converge at the jugular foramen and fuse in the large jugular ganglion. The glossopharyngeal nerve branches off immediately distal to the ganglion, the vagal and accessory fibers run in one bundle to the periphery, and the accessory nerve forms the second branch of the vagal nerve (Gaupp 1899).

In reptiles, the accessory nerve is either one of the branches of the vagal nerve and originates in a similar manner as in the frog or it emerges with a long caudal root from the cervical spinal cord and joins the vagus at the jugular foramen. Haller von Hallerstein (1934) describes variations, without reference to the species, in which an external and internal ramus can be distinguished. The former leaves the spinal canal with, or at the site of, the first cervical nerve. The internal ramus joins the vagal rootlets. In such cases this ramus carries the most caudal vagal fibers.

In most mammals the glossopharyngeal and vagal rootlets converge separately onto the jugular foramen and leave the braincase as two independent nerves. After a short intervening gap, a few caudal rootlets constitute the internal ramus of the accessory nerve which carries the most caudal vagal fibers. After a somewhat longer gap but along the same line, the roots of the spinal accessorius, or the ramus externus, emerge. As a rule, the bulbar and spinal accessorius merge as they enter the occipital foramen, then a communicating branch, the ramus internus, branches off and joins the vagal stem in the jugular foramen. The ramus internus innervates the muscles of the larynx, whereas the ramus externus is the nerve of the sternocleidomastoideus and trapezius muscles (Du Bois and Foley 1936; Romanes 1940).

9.3 The Topography and Cytoarchitecture of the Accessory Nerve Nucleus

9.3.1 Frog

When the vagal nerve is filled with cobalt, a few elongated polygonal neurons can be seen to be dispersed at the ventrolateral aspect of the ambiguus nucleus and discerned from vagal neurons by their larger size. In the medullospinal junction, where the ambiguus nucleus terminates, these neurons form a distinct group which extends as far caudally as the second spinal cord segment. They present ovoid or elongated polygonal perikarya measuring 30–50 μm in the longer diameter. (Fig. 15a). The dendritic arbor is oriented in the ventrolateral-dorsomedial direction in the obex region, and in the lateromedial direction in the spinal cord. The axons arise from the lateral dendrites, pull out into he lateral funiculus, and form a compact bundle of ascending fibers. Axons of more rostral neurons join this bundle which forms a root and merges with the vagal nerve at the medullospinal border.

On the basis of this finding we (Matesz and Székely 1978) have proposed for the first time that frogs have a spinal accessory nucleus (nXI) similar to that described in mammals. On the basis of their morphology and location, the accessory nerve neurons can be clearly distinguished from vagal neurons. Although according to the peripheral branching pattern the accessory nerve appears to be an adventitious part of the vagal nerve, its nucleus is entirely independent of the ambiguus nucleus. This proposition was corroborated in later experiments in which the accessory nerve proper, which supplies the cucullaris muscle, is labeled (Oka et al. 1987a; Matesz unpublished work). A comparable result was obtained in a number of salamander species by Roth et al. (1988) and Wake et al. (1988), including the ascending intramedullar bundle of axons of spinal accessory neurons. The existence of a mammalian type of nXI can, therefore, be generalized for amphibian species.

9.3.2 Lizard

If the common vagal-accessory nerve is labeled with cobalt, a new type of neuron appears in the rostral part of the spinal cord, about 200 μm caudal to the termination of the ambiguus nucleus. The elongated perikarya of these neurons are larger (40 μm) than the largest vagal neurons. A short medial and a long richly arborizing lateral dendritic arbor arises from the cell body (Fig. 15b). The lateral dendrites often give rise to a dorsally arching branch which lends the appearance of a general dorsolateral orientation to the lateral dendritic array. Otherwise, the arborization of the lateral dendrites resembles the broom-like pattern as seen in neurons of the branchiomotor nuclei. The axon emerges from the dorsomedial aspect of the neuron, runs to the mlf, and makes a sharp turn in the dorsolateral direction. The labeled fibers ascend intramedullary in the lateral funiculus, leave the spinal cord in two to three small rootlets, and the common root joins the vagal nerve in the jugular foramen (Székely and Matesz 1988).

This group of neurons clearly represents the nXI. Although the morphology of these neurons resembles that of other neurons in the ventrolateral motor column, they can be unambiguously distinguished from vagal neurons on account of their different size and location.

Following HRP application to the accessory nerve, labeled neurons were found in the first and second spinal cord segments by Barbas-Henry and Lohman (1984) in the *Anolis* lizard. They have interpreted their findings as showing that the ambiguus nucleus extended deep in the spinal cord representing the bulbar part of the nXI. They have admitted the possibility that a few neurons observed in the ventral horn of the first and second spinal cord segments might represent the spinal accessory origin of the vagal nerve. This ambiguous interpretation may have been influenced by the old view that a spinal component of the accessory nerve could not be identified in reptiles (Willard 1915).

9.3.3 Rat

The joint labeling of vagal and accessory nerves with cobalt reveals a long gap between the two nuclei of origin and a distinct difference in the morphology between the ambiguus and accessory nerve motoneurons. As described above, the ambiguus nucleus terminates where the pyramidal decussation begins. The next labeled neuron is encountered after a gap of about 1000 μm. The pyramidal decussation is nearly complete at this level. This is the rostral pole of the nXI, and the first neurons are found in the medial part of the ventral horn forming a medial column in the C1–C2 spinal cord segments. Before this column terminates it is adjoined by the lateral column of accessory nerve neurons which lies in the ventrolateral part of the ventral horn, and extends caudally as far as the sixth cervical segment. A few interposed cells are seen in the caudal part of C2.

The accessory nerve motoneurons are much bigger and show only some of the morphological features characteristic of ambiguus motoneurons. The polygonal perikarya are comparable in size to spinal motoneurons measuring 50–60 µm in diameter (Fig. 15c). Four to eight primary dendrites originate from the soma, and they are arranged in an irregular cross-shaped formation. The long limb of the cross is oriented in a dorsomedial-ventrolateral direction, the terminal twigs of the dorsomedial dendrites extend as far as the central canal. The ventrolateral dendritic arborization resembles the broom-shaped pattern of the ambiguus neurons. The axon invariably arises from the dorsal part of the perikaryon and takes a dorsally arched course between the ventral and dorsal horns toward the lateral aspect of the spinal cord. The rootlets emerge between the sensory and the motor rootlets of spinal nerves. In lower segments, many axons ascend for a distance of two to three segments in the lateral funiculus before entering the accessory rootlets.

This localization of the accessory nerve motoneurons which we (Matesz and Székely 1983) have obtained by cobalt labeling exactly corresponds to that found by Kitamura and Sakai (1982) and by Krammer et al. (1987) in the rat, and by Rapaport (1978) and Satomi et al. (1985) in the cat by HRP labeling. By injecting HRP into each of the five subdivisions of the rat sternocleidomastoideus and trapezius muscles, they have found a precise rostrocaudal representation of the sternomastoid, cleidomastoid, clavitrapezius, acromiotrapezius, and spinotrapezius muscles in the order listed. In addition to the accessorius motoneurons, a ventral cell group also contributes to the innervation of the last four muscle subdivisions. Axons of these neurons leave the spinal cord by way of the second through fourth ventral roots in an arrangement recognized in the early literature (Romanes 1940).

9.3.4 Conclusion

Our observations and the findings in a number of recent investigations clearly indicate the existence of the "spinal" accessory nerve and nucleus in lower vertebrates as well. Considering the conspicuous morphological differences, especially in the size between vagal and accessory nerve motoneurons, the latter is not a satellite structure of the former, but an independent nerve. As mentioned above, the first structure which can be regarded as the primordium of the trapezius-sternocleidomastoideus complex differentiates from the last gill arch elevator as the shoulder girdle appears in teleost fishes. This piece of muscle receives a branch from the vagal nerve. In amphibia, the muscles of gill arches are replaced by the four pharyngeal (petrohyoidei) muscles, and the fifth muscle becomes the cucullaris which is clearly separated from the last petrohyoideus muscle. Correspondingly, the separation of the accessory nerve and nucleus can be recognized in the frog. The independent nature of the accessory nerve and nucleus can be convincingly shown in higher vertebrates.

The reason why the idea of the bulbar accessory nerve persists in the modern literature may be found in the gross anatomical features of the origin of the nerve. As described above, the most caudal vagal roots derive from the loose formation of the ambiguus nucleus. They constitute the internal ramus of the accessory nerve. This branch, however, rejoins the vagal nerve at the jugular foramen and innervates the larynx (Du Bois and Foley 1936, Romanes 1940). This clearly indicates that the so-called bulbar accessory nerve represents the caudal part of the vagal nerve, consequently there is only a *spinal* accessory nerve.

If the accessory nerve originates in the spinal cord then the question emerges whether it is a cranial nerve or a spinal nerve, as suggested by Addens (1933). The evolution of the trapezius and sternocleidomastoideus muscles is suggestive of their origin from the primordial constrictor muscle from which muscles of the branchial arches derived. As shown above, these muscles are innervated by the ventrolateral motor column. The sternocleidomastoideus and trapezius muscles originate, at least partly, from the most caudal part of the primordial constrictor, and they became innervated by the most caudal part of the ventrolateral motoneurons of the medulla. Although these caudal neurons of the ventrolateral motor column are intermingled with spinal motoneurons, on the basis of their morphology (the dorsally arching axonal trajectory and the arborization pattern of dendrites) they can be clearly distinguished and compared to neurons of the rostral part of the ventrolateral motor column. According to these criteria the accessory nerve is a cranial nerve; but with the evolution of the cervical section of the spinal cord the accessory nerve motoneurons might have become trapped among spinal motoneurons and dragged in the caudal direction as the spinal cord gradually elongated. The long ascending axonal trajectory, whether intramedullary or extramedullary, is suggestive of this caudal shift of accessory nerve neurons. Thus, the spinal nXI is a detached and independent cranial nerve nucleus.

10 Neurons of the Cranial Parasympathetic Outflow

Despite the large number of investigations, relatively few reliable data are available about the brain stem parasympathetic preganglionic nuclei. Descriptions based on anatomical and physiological evidence are rather contradictory, even in mammals, ranging from discrete nuclei to a diffuse continuum of neurons scattered within the reticular formation. One of the reasons for the many contradictory results may be the poorly segregated nuclei of vegetative neurons as compared to rhabdomotor neurons. Another is the small size of the neurons and their thin axons which transport different tracer materials less readily. Since the brain stem vegetative system is most clearly explored in mammals, we describe first the rat parasympathetic neurons and compare these data with the results obtained from other species. In addition to our observations made on the lizard and the frog, we rely on the excellent descriptions by Contreras et al. (1980) in rats and by Reiner et al. (1983) in birds.

10.1 The Edinger-Westphal Nucleus and Ciliary Ganglion System

10.1.1 The Periphery

The ciliary ganglion can be dissected in most mammals used for laboratory work except the albino rat. The ganglion cannot be dissected in amphibia, but in some teleost fish it can be located on the inferior ramus of the ophthalmic nerve (Haller von Hallerstein 1934; Wathey 1988).

The periphery innervated by postganglionic fibers is primarily concerned with accommodation. This function is accomplished with different mechanisms in various animal species ranging from changing the position of the lens in fishes, amphibia, and ophidia to changing the curvature and thus the diopter of the lens in amniotes (Starck 1982). In this latter case, accommodation is accompanied by a reflexive pupilloconstriction which compensates for the increase in spherical aberration and the loss in depth of field that occur when the lens is in an accommodated state. Smooth muscle tissue implements this function, except the striated ciliaris muscle of sauropsidia. In birds, the ciliary ganglion also provides the parasympathetic innervation of smooth muscles of the choroidal coat of the eye serving to increase the choriocapillary blood flow by a vasodilatatory action on the choroidal arteries (Parver et al. 1982). The choroidal neurons receive boutonal endings whereas the ciliary neurons are contacted by so called calyciform endings suggesting a 1:1 pre- and postganglionic fiber relation (Pilar and Tuttle 1982). In the avian ciliary ganglion more than one half of neurons innervate the choroidal coat (Reiner et al. 1983). In the monkey, 3% of the neurons supply the iris sphincter, the rest innervates the ciliary body (Warwick 1954). In addition to the usual cholinergic transmission, preganglionic fibers contain substance P and enkephalin (Erichsen et al. 1982).

10.1.2 The Central Nucleus

Since the first description by Edinger (1885) and Westphal (1887), a very large body of data has been collected on the location and function of this visceral nucleus which bears the names of these authors. In view of the inconsistent terminology and the individual interpretation by the different authors, the exact definition of neuron groups which are concerned with the ciliary ganglion is very difficult. We try to specify the nuclei which are most often mentioned in relation to accommodation and pupilloconstriction on the basis of the descriptions by Olszewski and Baxter in humans (1954), and by Warwick (1954) and Carpenter and Peter (1970) in monkeys.

The Edinger-Westphal (EW) nucleus consists of a pair of slender columns of medium-sized neurons which dorsally overlie the main oculomotor nuclei. The two columns fuse in humans and arch over the rostral aspect of the oculomotor cell mass in a cap-like form. The ventral part of this cell group is generally denoted as the nucleus medianus anterior of Perlia. According to Akert et al. (1980), the cytoarchitecture of the nucleus medianus anterior and the EW nucleus distinctly differs from one another. The nucleus medianus anterior should not be confused with the nucleus of Perlia which is an unpaired centrally located cell group between the middle third of the oculomotor nuclei and used to be considered as being concerned with the control of convergence. As the paired EW nuclei extend caudally, they come to lie dorsomedial to the main oculomotor nuclei and dorsal to the nucleus of Perlia. This section of the visceral column is called also the dorsal visceral nucleus. Neurons in the medial part of the nucleus are larger than in the lateral part. The classic EW, therefore, consists of four subdivisions: the anterior median, and the dorsal, medial, and lateral visceral nuclei.

With the advent of modern tracing techniques a large number of contradictory results have been reported and have caused a great deal of confusion in the localization of the classically defined EW nuclear complex. The first source of confusion is the finding that the putative EW neurons project onto a variety of lower brain structures. In the spinal cord, EW fibers terminate in different laminae of the dorsal horn (Loewy and Saper 1978; Castiglioni et al. 1978; Carlton et al. 1985). Some of these fibers contain substance P and cholecystokinin (Maciewicz et al. 1983, 1984). In the brain stem, the cerebellum, the dorsal accessory olive, the parabrachial nucleus, the spinal trigeminal complex, and the dorsal column nuclei receive fibers from the area of the EW nucleus (Loewy and Saper 1978; Sugimoto et al. 1978; Maciewicz et al. 1984).

Another aspect of the contradictory results obtained from labeling experiments of the ciliary ganglion is the appearance of the tracer material outside the classically defined EW nuclear complex. While Akert et al. (1980) find the HRP label exclusively within the classic EW nucleus (except the anterior median nucleus) in monkeys (*Macaca fascicularis*), Burde and Loewy (1980) and Burde and Williams (1989) describe three distinct regions: the anterior median nucleus, the EW nucleus (as defined by Akert et al. 1980), and the nucleus of Perlia, all of which contain labeled neurons in the same monkey species. Preganglionic neurons which project to the ciliary ganglion are even more dispersed in the cat. Most of the labeled cells are encountered in the ventral tegmental area in the central gray matter in and around the anterior median nucleus but very few are found in the EW nucleus proper in the labeling experiments of Sugimoto et al. (1978), Toyoshima et al. (1980), and Maciewicz et al. (1983).

A brief conclusion that we can draw from these conflicting experiments concerning a general trend of organization is that the rostral part of the EW nucleus and the tegmental gray matter are mainly concerned with the ciliary ganglion, whereas the descending fibers originate mainly from the caudal part of the EW nucleus (Burde et al. 1982; Maciewicz et al. 1983). Both the ciliary and the descending contingents contain cholinergic and peptidergic (subtance P and cholecystokinin) neurons (Maciewicz et al. 1983, 1984; Strassman et al. 1987). These findings indicate that the region defined as the EW nuclear complex is much more delicate than a simple parasympathetic preganglionic nucleus. This has been already suggested by Szentágothai (1942) on the basis that the EW nucleus, in the strict classic sense, contains more than five times as many neurons as the ganglion ciliare.

The EW nucleus is a readily identifiable structure in birds. It is called the accessory oculomotor nucleus in early descriptions (Ariëns Kappers et al. 1936), and its relation to the ganglion ciliare is experimentally shown by Narayanan and Narayanan (1976). The avian EW nucleus is an elliptical group of cells above the dorsolateral subnucleus of the main oculomotor nucleus. A medial and a lateral subgroup can be discerned on a cytoarchitectonic basis, but functionally the nucleus is divided into three subdivisions (Reiner et al. 1983). Neurons in a narrow crescent area at the lateral margin of the nucleus are concerned with pupilloconstriction, the central part is occupied by neurons controlling accommodation, and a large medial subdivision subserves the choroidal vasodilatation.

A similar unambiguity can be found in the identification of the accessory oculomotor nucleus in reptiles (Ariëns Kappers et al. 1936), and its homology with the avian EW nucleus has been experimentally verified by Barbas-Henry and Lohman (1988) in the *Varanus* lizard. The nucleus occupies an oval-shaped area dorsal and lateral to the dorsal subnucleus in the rostral half of the main oculomotor nucleus.

There is only a single observation which gives account of an accessorius oculomotor nucleus in amphibia. Applying the cobalt label to the oculomotor root, Matesz and Székely (1978) mention the presence of a few labeled small neurons lying dorsal to the main oculomotor nucleus in the frog. Since the ganglion ciliare cannot be dissected in the frog, there is no experimental evidence for the ciliary relation of these neurons.

A homologue of the EW nucleus has recently been identified by retrograde labeling from the ciliary ganglion in teleost fishes (Wathey 1988). The small polygonal neurons can be seen dorsal and lateral to the main oculomotor nucleus at its rostral end. They extend laterally beyond the mlf.

10.2 The Medullary Parasympathetic Outflow

This system can be subdivided into a rostral and a caudal part. The first innervates glands and smooth muscles in the head region. The preganglionic efferent fibers are carried by branches of the facial and glossopharyngeal nerves to the periphery and terminate in one of the parasympathetic ganglia associated with the branches of the trigeminal nerve. The caudal part provides the parasympathetic innervation for thoracic and abdominal viscera. The preganglionic fibers are distributed by the vagal nerve and they terminate in the so-called intramural ganglia of the respective viscus.

10.2.1 The Peripheral Targets

Although the segregation of secretory cells to form multicellular glands can be observed in fishes, encapsulated salivatory glands of the oral cavity appear first in amphibia.These include a number of lingual and sublingual glands, palatine glands, and labial glands. In reptiles and birds, the glands are present in the form of glandular fields of secretory units rather than individual encapsulated glandular organs. Mammals have the three big salivary glands: the sublingual, submaxillary, and parotid glands, and there are numerous solitary and aggregated secretory units in the mouth and the pharynx (Fahrenholz 1937).

Lacrimal glands occur first in amphibia: the medial lacrimal gland or Harder's gland. This turns into the gland of the nictitating membrane in reptiles and birds, and the lateral, or true, lacrimal gland appears in these animals. Harder's gland is variously developed in different mammals; it is absent in some species, well developed and produces an oily secretion in aquatic mammals. The lateral lacrimal gland is usually well developed except for in Cetacea in which it is repressed (Starck 1982).

Very little is known about the parasympathetic supply of the vascular smooth muscle in the head region. In mammals, the choroid coat of the eye bulb is innervated by the postganglionic fibers of the sphenopalatine ganglion (Ruskel 1971).

Parasympathetic ganglia cannot be dissected in amphibia. The sphenopalatine and submandibular ganglia are present in reptiles and birds associated with the maxillary and lingual nerves, respectively. For details on the pre- and postganglionic relations the reader is referred to neuroanatomy textbooks.

10.2.2 The Distribution of the Preganglionic Neurons

Textbooks usually give account of well defined lacrimal and salivatory nuclei associated with branchial motor nuclei and of the dorsal motor nucleus of the vagal nerve (ndmX) which, due to the clear aggregation of its constituent neurons, is consistently defined in the early descriptions. Recent works, however, are more in favor of the view that most of the secretory preganglionic neurons are scattered in the parvicellular part of the reticular formation, and neurons of thoracic and abdominal viscera are aggregated in the ndmX. In addition to our cobalt studies on rats, lizards, and frogs, in the present description we rely on the excellent studies of Contreras et al. (1980) and Bieger and Hopkins (1987) on rats. Using HRP for retrograde labeling, their results are in good agreement with our results obtained from cobalt labeling experiments and also with a number of early observations.

10.2.2.1 Rat

The most rostral preganglionic neurons can be found at the level of the caudal one fourth of the facial genu scattered between this structure and the nucleus of the trapezoid body. These are middle-sized neurons, 20–30 μm in diameter. Many of them lie along the medial aspect of the descending limb of the facial root, the smaller cells situated dorsal to larger ones (Fig. 16a,b). There are two more or less distinct conglomerates formed by these cells, a ventral group is at the lateral aspect of the rostral pole of the nVIIm, and a smaller dorsal group is at the bend of the facial root (Fig. 16a). This level coincides with the caudal pole of the nVIIa.

A little more caudally, at the rostral tip of the nucleus of the solitary tract, another conglomerate of small cells 8–14 μm in diameter appears. These neurons are of the same size and form as the ndmX neurons and can be regarded as the most rostral extension of this nucleus. At about the same level but ventral to the rostral extension of the ndmX, a number of medium-sized neurons are scattered in the small-celled part of the reticular formation. The dorsal group of small cells (ndmX) and the field of scattered medium-sized neurons persist at the middle level of the facial nucleus. Here the number of

Fig. 16a–g. Parasympathetic preganglionic neurons in the rat medulla oblongata. **a** Lateral view of the medulla indicating the topographical distribution of preganglionic neurons. At the rostral pole of the VIIm and subjacent to the rostral end of the dorsal motor nucleus of the vagus (*dmX*), three relatively well defined conglomerates are outlined; the localization of the scattered neurons are shown by *small circles*; *arrows* indicate the sites of subjacent photographs with identical letters. **b** Small neurons at the caudal pole of the nVIIa. *Arrow with bar* indicates the arching course of axons of these neurons as they join the axon bundle of the nVIIa (*arrow*); *Asterisks* show the ascending limb of the root of the nVIIm. **c** Camera lucida reconstruction of a relatively large neuron at the medial aspect of the descending limb of the facial root. Note the ascending axon (*arrow*). In **b**, **c** the facial nerve was labeled with cobalt. **d** Three groups of cells are shown at the rostral pole of the ambiguus nucleus after labeling the glossopharyngeal nerve. The small cells of the dmX are in the *right upper corner*; the medium-sized cells are framed with a *broken line*; the large ventrolateral cells are in the *left lower corner*. The same groups of neurons are outlined in **a**, **e**, **f**, **g**, where the vagal nerve was labeled. In **e** the dmX is shown in the obex region. In **f** a solitary neuron is seen in the external formation of the ambiguus nucleus. *Arrows* indicate the vagal root. In **g** small neurons are indicated by *arrows* lateral to the large cells of the loose formation of the ambiguus nucleus. *Calibration bar* is 50 μm in **e**; 100 μm in **b**, **c**, **f**, **g** ▷

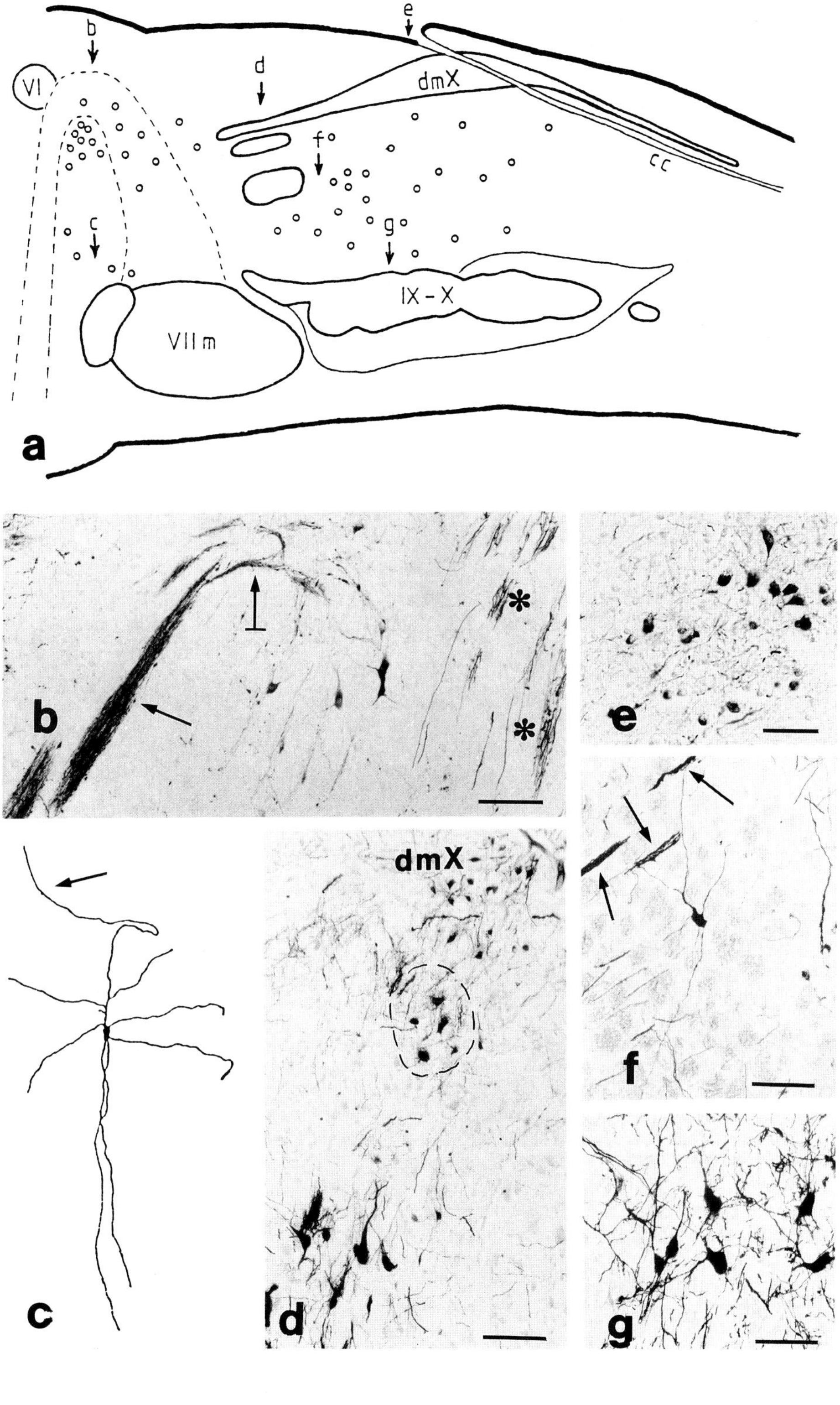

VI
b
e
d
dmX
f
cc
c
g
IX-X
VIIm
a
b
e
f
dmX
c
d
g

small neurons increases in the ndmX, and the majority of the scattered neurons conglomerate and form two globular accumulations ventral and lateral to the dorsal group (Fig. 16a,d). Neurons are segregated in such a manner that the most ventral group consists of large neurons (20–25 µm) whereas the group lying midway between this and the ndmX consists of medium-sized (15–20 µm) cells.

A little more caudally, at the rostral pole of the ambiguus nucleus, the ndmX together with the solitary tract and nucleus shifts medially and occupies its position classically defined (Fig. 16e). The number of neurons continues to increase in this dorsomedial position and the ndmX extends caudally into the cervical spinal cord as far as the rostral pole of the nXI. A few medium-sized neurons occur scattered between the ambiguus nucleus and the ndmX, and they can be followed almost to the caudal pole of the ambiguus nucleus although in smaller numbers than at more rostral levels (Fig. 16f). An appreciable number of middle-sized neurons can be found within, lateral and ventral to the ambiguus nucleus (Fig. 16g) and corresponding to the external formation of this nucleus (Hopkins 1987).

From the globular or spindle-shaped perikarya two to four dendrites emerge and often occupy a dorsoventral orientation. The axon invariably originates from the dorsal aspect of the perikaryon, runs in the dorsomedial direction to different distances, arches ventrolaterally, and joins one of the rootlets of the facial, glossopharyngeal, and vagal nerves (Fig. 16b,c).

10.2.2.2 Lizard

The distribution of a contingent of small and medium-sized neurons, which can be labeled from the facial, glossopharyngeal, and vagal nerves, is very similar to that described for the rat; however, the conglomeration of the scattered neurons into distinct groups is less conspicuous. As described in our earlier paper (Székely and Matesz 1988), the nVII consists of a medial large-celled and a lateral small-celled group of neurons. The former is a group of morphologically homogeneous neurons which innervate branchiogenous

Fig. 17a–g. Parasympathetic preganglionic neurons in the medulla oblongata. **a–d** Lizard. ▷ In **a** the facial nerve was labeled. *Dotted line* demarcates the most rostral extension of the dorsal motor nucleus of the vagus; (dmX) *arrows* point at neurons "scattered" between the nVII and dmX. *Arrows with bar* indicate the dorsomedially ascending axons. In **b** the glossopharyngeal nerve was filled. The dmX is outlined ventral to the solitary tract and nucleus (*SOL*). Arrows point at the "scattered" neurons. On the right margin the 4th ventricle is seen (4th). In **c**, **d** the vagal nerve was filled. The dmX is outlined in the obex region and in the medullospinal junction. *Cc*, the central canal. The larger labeled cells represent the nX and the unlabeled large neurons the nXII. **e–g** Frog. In **e** the facial nerve was labeled. The presumably preganglionic neurons are *circled*. The *arrow* points at their axons joining the solitary tract (*SOL*). In **f** the glossopharyngeal nerve was labeled. *Arrows* point at small, presumably preganglionic, neurons lying dorsal to nIX. Their axons (*arrow with bar*) take a separate course and join the solitary tract. In **g** the vagal nerve was labeled. Two small neurons (*circled*) represent the presumably dmX dorsal to the nX. *Calibration bar* is 100 µm

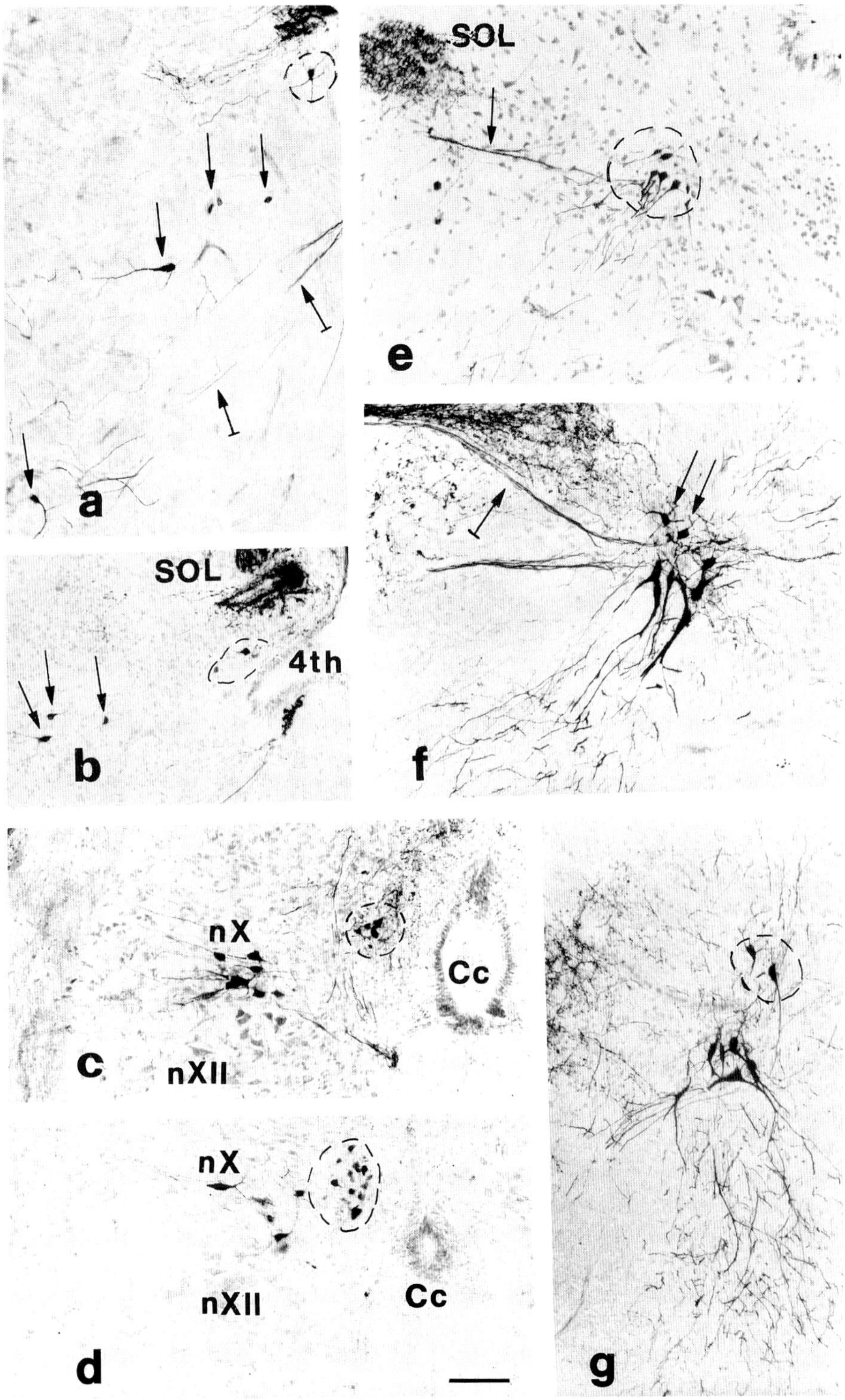
SOL
a
SOL
4th
b
nX
Cc
c
nXII
nX
nXII
Cc
d
e
f
g

muscles, whereas the small size (15–17 μm) and the morphological heterogeneity suggest the visceromotor nature of neurons in the lateral group. At the same level with the facial nuclear complex, a number of small neurons form a compact column ventral to the solitary tract. This is clearly the rostral extension of the ndmX (Fig. 17a). A third group of neurons can be found scattered in the reticular formation between the lateral subnucleus of the nVII and the ndmX (Fig. 17a,b). Their size gradually decreases from the ventral to the dorsal direction.

The nIX is fused with the nVII and the presumably parasympathetic neurons continue in a scattered arrangement down to the obex region in the reticular formation. The dorsomedial cell column, the ndmX, continues caudally in the classical site (Fig. 17c), and its caudal end extends into the medullospinal junction below the level of the commissura infima (Fig. 17d). Scattered neurons can be found also in the lateral part of the medullary reticular formation at the level of the nXII. Their axons run in the vagal nerve. A common morphological feature of all these neurons is that their axons emerge from the dorsal aspect of the somata, course toward the mlf, make a hairpin turn, and join the roots of the facial, glossopharyngeal, and vagal nerves (Székely and Matesz 1988).

10.2.2.3 Frog

With cobalt labeling of the facial nerve a group of small neurons (14–18 μm) are stained at the level of the abducens nucleus in the dorsolateral part of the gray matter (Matesz and Székely 1978). The dendritic arbor is oriented in the dorsoventral direction, the axon arises from the lateral dendrite, joins the afferent fibers of the facial nerve, and leaves the medulla through the intermedius nerve (Fig. 17e).

The ndmX is only partially segregated in amphibia (Fig. 17f,g). However, small cells of similar shape can be found at the dorsal aspect of both the nIX and nX more or less separated from the large motor neurons of these nuclei (Matesz and Székely 1978; Oka et al. 1987b; Matesz unpublished).

10.2.3 The Organization of the Medullary Preganglionic Neurons

Experimental studies on the distribution of preganglionic neurons innervating different viscera have been done only in mammalian species. We can make only some inferences that, in the frog, the small group of neurons which send axons through the facial nerve may innervate Harder's gland and the intermaxillary glands, and the small neurons in the nIX and nX may be homologues of the ndmX. The distribution of the allegedly preganglionic neurons of the lizard is very similar to that of the rat, and the scheme of organization that we detail below for the rat probably applies to the lizard as well.

The best data on the organization of the parasympathetic preganglionic neurons belonging to the facial and glossopharyngeal nerves of the rat can be found in the work of Contreras et al. (1980). The ventral group of neurons situated rostral and lateral to the nVIIm send axons to the sphenopalatine ganglion by way of the greater superficial petrosal nerve. Neurons which are scattered in the parvicellular reticular formation between the nVIIm and the genu and the conglomerate of medium and large neurons ventral to the ndmX may be regarded as the main salivatory "center" since the axons reach the submaxillary and otic ganglia from this area. The most dorsal of these neurons, which are the smallest, form a small group medial to the nucleus of the solitary tract constituting the rostral tip of the classically defined ndmX. Neurons in the rostral one fourth of this column and the medium-sized neurons send their axons to the lingual branch of the glossopharyngeal nerve supplying serous glands which flush the moatlike trough around the taste papillae of the tongue.

Caudal to the level of the posterior pole of the nVIIm, neurons of the ndmX send their axons to the vagal nerve and innervate thoracic and abdominal viscera. While efferent neurons which innervate the mucous membrane of the esophagus are localized in the rostral one third of the vagal section of the ndmX in the dog (Hudson and Cummings 1985), a somatotopic representation is not apparent for other viscera innervated by the vagal nerve. Other authors maintain that individual subdiaphragmatic branches of the vagal nerve are represented in longitudinal columns in the ndmX (Prechtl and Powley 1985). In contrast to these findings in mammals, a clear subnuclear heterogeneity is found in the pigeon ndmX which discloses a well defined topographic organ representation (Katz and Karten 1983). In this respect the vagal section of the nucleus can be divided in a rostral part anterior to the obex and a caudal part. In the rostral part there is a rostrocaudal sequence in the representation of the cervical esophagus, thoracic esophagus, and the glandular stomach. In the caudal part of the nucleus the sequence of this visceral representation is reversed.

The innervation of the heart originates from a group of medium-sized neurons located at the ventrolateral aspect of the ambiguus nucleus, called the external formation, and there is only a minor contribution from the dorsal motor nucleus. This has been shown in a variety of animals including the rat (Nosaka et al. 1979; Stuesse 1982), the cat (Ciriello and Calaresu 1982), the dog (Hopkins and Armour 1982), and the pig (Hopkins et al. 1984). In addition to this ventrolateral cell group, neurons of similar size and shape are dispersed among the large cells of the ambiguus nucleus (Fig. 16g). Their locations correspond to the representation of the heart innervation described in the above works. The mixing of the large and medium-sized neurons might have been the background of the confusion about the "specific" and "general" efferent nature of the ambiguus nucleus in old descriptions.

10.3 Conclusion

According to their positions the parasympathetic preganglionic neurons can be classified into a mesencephalic and a medullary division. The mesencephalic division is represented by the EW nucleus. In contrast to the classic view, the parasympathetic neurons do not form a compact nucleus but they are dispersed in the central gray matter intermingled with a number of interneurons with descending and ascending projections. While this is the situation in all mammals investigated, the classic EW nucleus is present in reptile and birds. The almost complete segregation of the presynaptic neurons and the one to one relation of the preganglionic and postganglionic fibers in the ciliary ganglion (Szentágothai 1942) and striated muscle in the ciliary body suggest a high level of differentiation of the ciliary system in these animals which are primarily dependent on vision.

In the medullary division there is only one cluster of neurons which can be unambiguously defined as a nucleus, that is, the dorsal motor nucleus of the vagus. It extends, however, rostrally to a much greater extent than classically defined. This nucleus consists of very small neurons, the smallest efferent neurons in the nervous system, which are fairly homogeneous in shape and size. The axons enter the facial, glossopharyngeal, and vagal nerves; it seems, therefore, to be more appropriate to call this group of neurons the *dorsal visceromotor column of the medulla*.

A strict regularity cannot be recognized in the distribution of the rest of the preganglionic neurons. They are mainly scattered in the parvicellular part of the reticular formation between the dorsal visceromotor column and the ventrolateral branchiomotor column coexistent rostrocaudally with the former in the parvicellular part of the reticular formation. The neurons are of variable size and secretomotor and vasomotor cells cannot be distinguished from one another. The neurons may form smaller or larger aggregates in various sites in different species. The most stable formations seem to be the group lateral to the facial nucleus, which belongs to the facial nerve, and the group dorsal to the facial nucleus, which belongs to the glossopharyngeal nerve. We think that instead of calling these variously compact formation nuclei, the part of the reticular formation containing preganglionic neurons may be designated as the *lateral visceromotor area of the medulla*.

There are a number of medium-sized neurons around and within the vagal part of the ambiguus nucleus. Tracer studies have shown that they innervate the heart. Due to their smaller size and the fewer number of dendrites, these neurons can be distinguished from the larger ones which innervate branchiogenous striated muscles. Thus the visceral and the branchiomotor parts can be clearly distinguished and this makes the ambiguus nucleus less ambiguous.

11 General Conclusions

Our work has been initiated by a number of misconceptions about the structure of the cranial nerve nuclei. Despite many recent findings in disagreement with the old concepts, these misconceptions survive in modern textbooks and cause many problems in comprehending the efferent outflow of the brainstem. We have approached these problems with a twofold stratagy. First, we have relied on the neural morphology in sorting out the different groups of nerve cells; second, we have done this on three distantly related animal species in order to compare the interspecies similarities and diversities. The double approach has its vulnerability. A voluntarist interpretation of the neural morphology may result in arbitrary groupings of neurons according to some preconceived view. We have been continuously aware of this possibility and have tried to be very careful about interspecies similarities or diversities. Second, using the data obtained only from three species for a comparative neuroanatomy study is like tiptoeing from tussock to tussock over a marshy field. Here we have also been aware of the danger of slipping into new misconceptions however carefully we proceed. The probable gaps should be filled and the misconceptions corrected in future works, but a few basic principles and some inferences may be offered from the present work as well.

11.1 The Arrangement of Cranial Nerve Motor Nuclei

Figure 18 summarizes our findings on the organization of cranial nerve motor nuclei. It is clear at the first sight that there are more than just two columns of motoneurons even in the frog brain stem, and the old classification is an oversimplification. Starting from the midline and proceeding in an onion peel-like manner toward the surface, we can distinguish the following nuclear groups:

1. As far as their position and organization are concerned, the eye moving motoneurons constitute the most conservative nuclear group. They are next to the midline, interconnected by the mlf; the musculotopic representation and the emergence of the nerves are remarkably stable in all vertebrate species. One is tempted to venture the notion that no better solution can be conceived for the movement of a globe in all possible directions than the four recti and the two obliqui muscles.
2. The conspicuously characteristic neuronal morphology throughout the different species clearly distinguishes the other dorsomedial nucleus from the

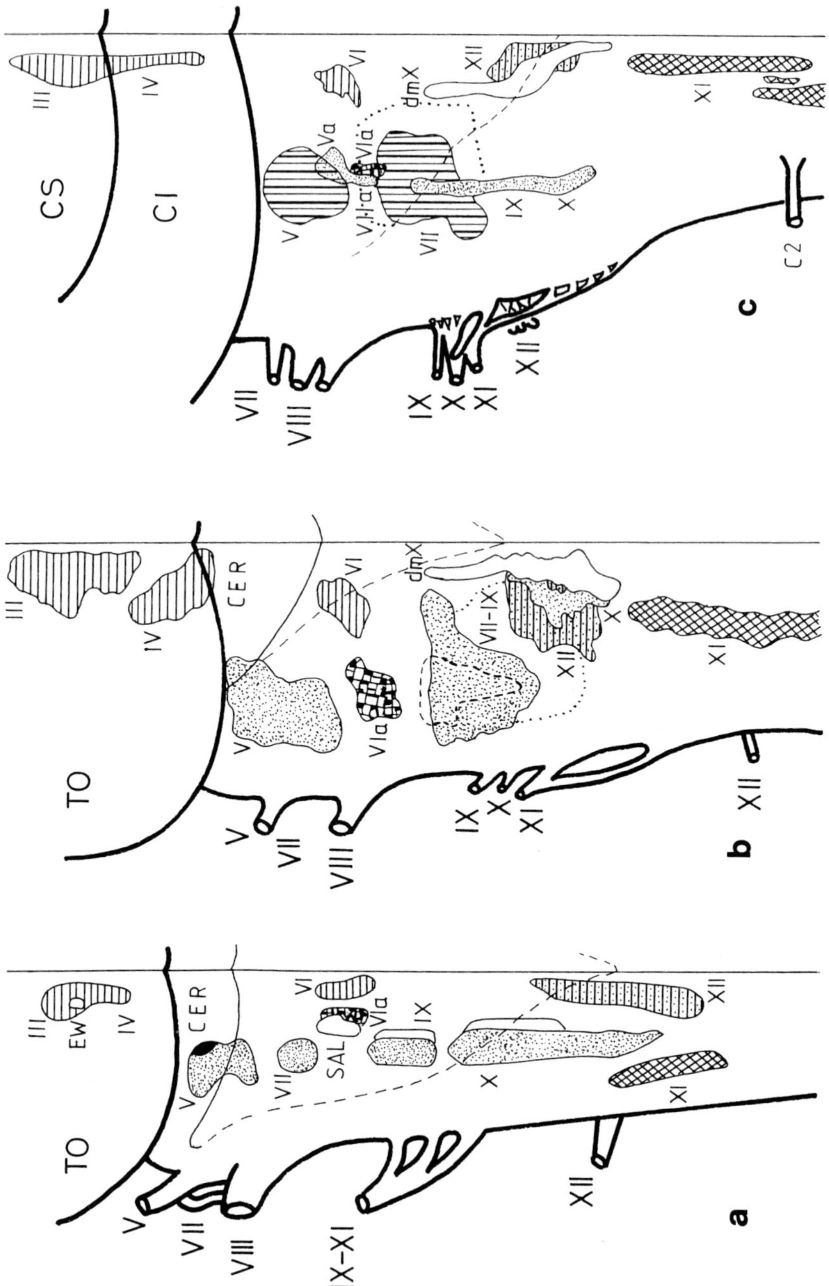

Fig. 18a–c. Dorsal view of the topography of cranial nerve nuclei in the frog (**a**), lizard (**b**), and rat (**c**). The sizes are greatly distorted for the sake of a joint representation of the three brain stems. *Roman numerals* indicate the respective roots and nuclei. *TO*, optic tectum; *CS* and *CI*, superior and inferior colliculi; *EW*, Edinger-Westphal nucleus (*empty area*); *CER*, cerebellum; *SAL*, superior salivatory nucleus. Note that the different nuclear columns are identified by different patterns. Nuclei of the external eye muscles are *horizontally hatched*; the hypoglossal nuclei are *hatched* and *stippled*; the accessory abducens nuclei are *checkered*; the branchiomotor columns are *stippled* (note the nVa and nVIIa are in this group);

eye moving motor nuclei. The nXII is a relatively novel structure which is found first in tetrapods with a muscular tongue. The nucleus is at the medullospinal transition intermingled, though in a distinguishable manner, with motoneurons of some of the hyoid muscles. The position and the intermingling of its neurons may have caused the confusion about the hypoglossal nucleus in the old literature.

3. The mechanism of eye withdrawal controlled by the nVIa is also a novel structure appearing first in tetrapods. Its lateral position induced some speculation about "neurobiotaxis" which could not be corroborated in recent experiments (Matesz 1990a). In a teleological way of thinking, the acquisition of the retractor bulbi muscles and the corresponding neural apparatus basically contributed to the capability of land living. Curiously enough, this mechanism disappeared in apes and human.
4. The levator bulbi muscle and the innervating motoneurons incorporated in the nV is a peculiar structure in amphibia. We could not find a comparable structure in the lizard, perhaps the depressor of the inferior eyelid of birds may be its homologue. The smooth orbital muscle with sympathetic innervation is erroneously held as the homologue of the levator bulbi.
5. Parallel to the differentiation of the rostral region of animals, neurons controlling the movements of the mouth and gills disclose the largest scale of changes in phylogenesis. Unfortunately, we do not have sufficient data to include the fish brain in this discussion; still, tremendous changes can be observed just in the three species investigated. On a neuromorphological basis, we could clearly distinguish jaw closer and opener neurons in the nV and nVII of the frog. The opener type of neuron is also found in the nIX and nX of this animal suggesting a common origin and perhaps related function of the muscles innervated by this type of neuron. It is possible to distinguish closer and opener neurons also in the lizard, and the latter type of neuron is found in the fused nVII and nIX, and a smaller variety of this type in the reduced nX. Therefore, the branchiomotor nuclei including the nV, nVII, nIX, and nX, form a well defined almost continuous column in submammalian vertebrates. In view of the spatial separation of nIX and nX, an ambiguus nucleus does not develop in these animals.
6. There are profound changes in the mammalian brain stem associated with the differentiation of the secondary jaw joint, the secondary palate, and the muscles of mastication and facial expression. The closer neurons are replaced by the masticatory neurons and they constitute the large nVm situated lateral to the nVa. The openers persist, form a common column of the nVa and nVIIa, and innervate the suprahyoid muscles. New type of neurons appear for the innervation of some pharyngopalatal muscles and the striated muscles of the esophagus, and these neurons connect the nIX and the nX forming the ambiguus nucleus which can unambiguously be

◁ **Fig. 18** (*continued*). the accessory nerve nuclei are *cross-hatched*; the *black spot* in the frog nV indicates levator bulbi neurons; the main trigeminal and facial nuclei are *vertically hatched* in the rat brain; the parasympathetic nuclei are *empty*; the area of "scattered" neurons is outlined by *dots* in the lizard and rat brains; the lateral facial subnucleus is indicated by *broken line* in the lizard brain distinguished only in mammals. The neuron population of the mammalian ambiguus nucleus is made heterogeneous by the presence of the large polygonal neurons which innervate the larynx. Therefore, in the mammal the primordial column of the branchial motor nuclei is constituted by the nVa, nVIIa, and the ambiguus nucleus, the latter with a heterogeneous neuron population. Lateral to this column are two novel structures: the nVm for mastication and the nVIIm for facial expression, and the presence of large polygonal neurons indicates the appearance of a new type of neuron in the ambiguus nucleus.

7. The innervation of the auditory muscles outside the traditionally assumed trigeminal and facial nuclei has been only recently recognized. These neurons form a continuous column in the most ventrolateral part of the entire length of the metencephalon.
8. The most caudal structure is the nXI which has no relation to the ambiguus nucleus. Its neurons are intermingled with vagal neurons in the frog, they are spatially separated in the lizard, and located entirely in the spinal cord (i.e., caudal to the pyramidal decussation) in the rat. We suggest that this caudal disposition may be the consequence of the elongation of the cervical section of the spinal cord.
9. The parasympathetic preganglionic neurons can be found in the mesencephalon associated with the nIII and in the medulla. In the latter site there is only a single well delineated group of neurons, the ndmX, which contributes to the facial, glossopharyngeal, and vagal nerves. In view of the wide extension of its field of innervation, this nucleus may be called the dorsal visceromotor column of the medulla. The rest of the preganglionic neurons are scattered or form small irregular groups in the parvicellular part of the bulbar reticular formation representing the lateral visceromotor area of the medulla.

11.2 Comments on the Morphological Classification

On the basis of their dendritic geometry and axonal trajectory, we have distinguished seven types of neurons. (1) The most numerous group is constituted by neurons innervating branchial structures. They are characterized by the dorsoventrally oriented dendritic tree and the dorsally looping axonal trajectory. These neurons are found mainly in a ventrolateral position constituting the primordial branchiomotor column. (2) Preganglionic neurons of similar type are scattered, or form more or less distinct aggregations, in the medulla. On the basis of the cell body and the dendritic arborization pattern, many subgroups can be discerned in this type, but the dorsally looping axonal trajectory is invariably present in all subgroups. In the midline, two different types can be clearly distinguished: (3) the eye moving neurons and (4) the tongue motoneurons. (5) Neurons innervating the retractor bulbi muscles clearly represent a separate type. (6) The levator bulbi neurons form a unique type which is present only in amphibia. (7) The large neurons in the mammalian trigeminal and facial nuclei also constitute an unambiguously distinguishable type. This latter type differs in a number of features from the other neurons and occupies the most lateral position in the hindbrain. The axons emerge from the ventral aspect of these neurons and run straight to the site of exit in the case of the trigeminus and to the facial genu in case of the facialis. In the facial genu axons form a long whirl-like structure lateral to the nVI before turning ventrally to the site of exit. The internal genu of the facial nerve is, therefore, distinctly different from the dorsal loops or hairpin turns of axons of the first and second types of neurons.

These seven types of neurons almost correspond to the eight groups of cranial nerve neurons, as we have classified them in the previous chapter, in which functionally identical or similar neuron pools are grouped together. This parallelism refers to a kind of form-function relationship. In fact, some of the neurons have such characteristic morphological features across the three species investigated that we can speak about hypoglossal neurons, accessory abducens neurons, and levator bulbi neurons. The closer and opener neurons can also be clearly distinguished from one another, and the opener type can be unambiguously recognized in the rat nVa and nVIIa. A similar conspicuous form-function relationship can be found in the spinal cord, in which motoneurons innervating limb muscles distinctly differ in their dendritic geometry from motoneurons which supply trunk muscles (Székely 1976). It would be difficult to explain the mechanisms by which form relates to function. One may refer to the different disposition and expansion of the postsynaptic receptive field by which neurons with different morphologies and position may be connected to different central apparatuses of the brain. The several examples of the common groups and columns formed by neurons controlling the same function are also suggestive of such a mechanism.

11.3 Trends in the Evolution of Cranial Nerve Nuclei

The classification of neurons on a morphological basis provides a unique possibility to follow their fate in the three species investigated and venture some surmises about possible changes in phylogenesis. While we do this, we are aware of the danger of making generalizations on the basis of data obtained from a limited number of species. The main question we want to discuss is whether the evolutionary trend in the field of cranial nerve nuclei is the transformation of preexisting structures or the acquisition of novel structures during phylogenesis. It is clear that no direct evidence can be found to support either of these evolutionary mechanisms; still, we would like to point out a few examples that we think are in favor of the latter alternative.

First, we want to refer to the rather conservative character of the eye moving motor nuclei which do not show much change except for the increasingly distinct musculotopic partition of the nuclear group in mammals. A similar conservatism can be seen in the innervation of the intrinsic tongue muscles, the characteristic hypoglossal form of neurons, which distinctly differs from spinal motoneurons and is preserved in the three species investigated. Not much change occurred in the periphery of these motor nuclei during phylogenesis.

Spectacular changes can be recorded in the structures of the branchial region. A discussion of the transition from the gill apparatus to lung breathing is not in the frame of the present endeavor, therefore we want to limit our consideration to the differences observed in the three species investigated. Muscles in the trigeminal and facial region of the frog and lizard are unanimously regarded as homologues in modern comparative anatomy (Starck 1982), and in fact the only difference is the richness in form and shape in the lizard mandibular apparatus as compared to the frog. It is very probable that this richness differentiated from preexisting material. The same event can be seen in the center. Muscles of the primary mandibular joint are innervated by the type 1 neurons which disclose a larger morphological variety in the lizard than in the frog. By the same token we may assume that the morphological richness of the type 1 neurons of the lizard differentiated from the basic form of the closer and opener type of neurons which is present and clearly distinguishable in the frog. If, however, something disappears from the periphery it also does from the center, for example, the levator bulbi muscle and its characteristic motoneurons are not found in the lizard.

Profound changes can be witnessed in the area of the trigeminal and facial nerves in the rat. The transformation of the primary mandibular joint involves the appearance of new structures including among others the mandible with gomphotic teeth and a new set of muscles which, according to Starck (1982), cannot be homologized with the closer muscles of lower vertebrates. For the sake of distinction we call them masticatory muscles. The suprahyoid muscle group, by contrast, can be derived from homologous counterparts of submammalian tetrapods. While the innervation of the suprahyoid muscle group originates from the opener type of neurons of the nVa and nVIIa, the closer type of neurons are not found in the trigeminal nucleus; they are replaced by the masticatory neurons constituting the nVm which lies lateral to the nVa-nVIIa complex. The dendritic geometry and axonal trajectory of the masticatory neurons are so profoundly different from the closer neurons that they probably represent a novel structure in the trigeminal nuclear complex.

A similar train of thought can be continued with respect to the mammalian facial nucleus which has no relation to the submammalian facial nerve. If we regard the nVIIm as a novel structure, then the muscles of facial expression are also a novel acquisition and cannot be derived from the sphincter colli as is generally maintained in the literature (see Chapt. 6). The heterogeneity of the neuron population of the mammalian ambiguus nucleus can also be the result of the appearance of new types of nerve cells which innervate novel structures in the vagus area, that is, muscles of the soft palate, the esophagus, and the larynx.

These few examples are in favor of the suggestion that some types of neurons disappear and others are newly acquired in the central nervous system during phylogenesis. The mechanism of these changes, whether they occur gradually, as generally maintained in the literature, or suddenly, as seen in our limited examples, remains concealed with the extinction of mammal-like reptiles and other transitory forms. We hope to obtain data for these problems from the study of the changes of cranial nerve nuclei in tadpoles during the metamorphic climax.

11.4 Corollary Considerations

As a corollary to the above surmises, we can touch upon two more problems presented often in comparative anatomy studies. The first is the problem of muscle homologies, the second is the question of head segmentation.

Muscle homologies are generally established on the basis of comparative anatomical observations supplemented by descriptive embryological studies on the origin of the muscle in question. Such descriptive accounts often resulted in erroneous conclusions, e.g., the homology of the superficial neck constrictor of reptiles with the mammalian platysma, or the classic misconception about the lateral plate origin of the branchial musculature. Noden's (1983) observation that all craniofacial muscles derive from the condensation of the paraxial mesoderm is a good warning against the unconditional application of embryological data to the problems of homology of some particular muscle groups. On the basis of our results we suggest that the form and site of the innervating nerve cells can provide important supplementary data for the establishment of homologies.

The problem of head segmentation is shortly mentioned in the Introduction. Whether the head consists of structural elements placed serially one after another or not implies the same question which we tackled in the previous chapter: did the head evolve from preexisting structures or it is a novel acquisition? Our findings that novel neural structures emerge during phylogenesis do not support the segmentation theory. Furthermore, since all craniofacial muscles derive from the segmented paraxial mesoderm and migrate secondarily to their final positions, there does not seem to be much sense in a tenacious effort to detect the preotic head segments, the vestigial traces of serial building elements of the head. The somatomotor and specific visceromotor distinction of craniofacial muscles also becomes meaningless in light of this mechanism of muscle development and innervation.

11.5 Summary

A number of inconsistencies and controversies are inherent in the classification of cranial nerve nuclei based on the concepts of the various head-theories. The assumption of head segmentation, which is common to these theories, serves as the basis for designating the dorsomedial nuclei as the somatomotor column, although they innervate striated muscles of a viscus and a specific sense organ. The ventrolateral nuclei are called the specific visceromotor column; they innervate striated muscles in the branchiogenous area, but many of these muscles insert on skeletal elements. A series of comparative neuromorphological studies investigating the dendritic arborization pattern and axonal trajectory in the frog, lizard, and rat suggests a much more delicate classification in which nine morphologically and functionally different neuron groups can be discerned:

1. The hypoglossal nucleus appears coincidentally with the muscular tongue in amphibia. The spindle-shaped perikaryon, the bipolar dendritic arboriza-

tion, and the straight ventral trajectory of the axon are characteristic morphological features in all three animal species investigated.

2. The oculomotor, trochlear, and abducens nuclei present a remarkably conservative topography and organization in all vertebrates with a moving eye. With their oval-shaped or polygonal perikarya and radiating dendritic arborization, these neurons distinctly differ from hypoglossal neurons. The ipsilateral axons follow a straight ventral course, the contralateral axons form a dorsal loop before crossing the midline, and the crossing is not consequence of neuron migration to the contralateral side.
3. The accessory abducens nucleus is present in tetrapods except apes and human. The elongated perikaryon and the dorsoventral dendritic orientation distinctly distinguish these neurons from other cranial motoneurons. the nucleus is found in the lateral part of the reticular formation. The neurons differentiate in situ, they do not migrate from the main abducens nucleus.
4. In the submammalian trigeminal and facial nuclei, two basic neuron types can be distinguished on the basis of their morphology. The first type is larger and accumulates in the rostral part of the trigeminal nucleus. This type innervates the jaw closer muscles. The second type is found in the caudal part of the trigeminal nucleus and in the facial nucleus. These neurons innervate the muscular floor of the mouth and the facial contingent supplies the jaw opener muscle. A very characteristic feature in the axonal trajectory is an initial medial course and a hairpin turn, or dorsal loop, at the lateral aspect of the medial longitudinal fasciculus. In addition to the two types of neurons, there is a third type in the frog trigeminal nucleus. This innervates an orbital muscle. This type of neuron and the muscle cannot be found in the lizard.
5. In the area of innervation of the mammalian trigeminal and facial nuclear complex, new structures develop, including the secondary temporomandibular joint, the masticatory muscles, the secondary palate and its muscles, and the muscles of facial expression. These changes render possible the act of mastication. The jaw closer neuron type is replaced by a morphologically different neuron type in the trigeminal nucleus which innervates the mammalian masticatory muscles. Medial and ventral to this neuron group, another type of neuron is found which exhibits a dendritic arborization and axonal trajectory similar to the second type of neuron in the submammalian trigeminal and facial nuclei. These neurons constitute the accessory trigeminal nucleus and innervate the muscular floor of the mouth and the anterior digastric muscle. The mammalian facial nucleus comprises a neuron type which is similar to the neurons of the main trigeminal nucleus. Axons of these neurons form the facial genu and innervate the muscles of facial expression. Dorsal to this neuron group, a second type of neuron forms the accessory facial nucleus. It is continuous with the accessory trigeminal nucleus and innervates the posterior digastric and the stylohyoideus muscles. The accessory trigeminal and facial nuclei represent their submammalian counterparts and supply muscles with the same function, whereas the main trigeminal and facial nuclei are new acquisitions and control new functions, mastication and facial expression, in mammalian species.

6. The neuron group supplying the auditory muscles forms a continuous column rostral to the facial nucleus and ventral to the trigeminal nucleus in the mammalian pontine tegmentum. The rostral neurons innervate the tensor tympani muscle via the trigeminal nerve, the caudal neurons innervate the stapedius muscle via the facial nerve.
7. The glossopharyngeal and vagal nuclear complex consists of two separate nuclei in the frog and the lizard. They contain a neuron type which is similar in form to the second type of neuron in the trigeminal and facial nuclei. The glossopharyngeal nucleus is fused with the facial nucleus, and the vagal nucleus is reduced in size in the lizard. In the mammalian medulla, a new type of neuron appears which innervates muscles of the soft palate and striated muscles of the esophagus. These neurons bridge the gap between the glossopharyngeal and vagal nuclei and the ambiguus nucleus is formed.
8. On the basis of neuronal morphology, the nucleus of the accessory nerve can be clearly distinguished from the vagal (ambiguus) nucleus. The accessory nerve nucleus is shifted caudally into the rostral spinal cord; it has no vagal component.
9. Preganglionic parasympathetic neurons are found in the mesencephalon, the EW nucleus, and in the medulla oblongata. In this latter part of the brain, two main neuron populations can be discerned. In one of them the neurons are dispersed in the lateral part of the reticular formation forming more or less defined aggregations in some places; These innervate the various salivatory glands. The second neuron population forms a distinct column in a dorsomedial position corresponding to the classically defined dorsal motor nucleus of the vagus. Axons of this nucleus contribute to the facial, glossopharyngeal, and vagal nerves.

On the basis of these findings it is concluded that changes in the periphery are accompanied by corresponding changes in the appropriate nerve centers during phylogenesis. In the course of these changes, some types of neurons disappear while new types appear bringing forth new functions. As a collorary, it is suggested that the type of innervation can provide useful directives in establishing homologies between muscle groups of different animal species and that the organization of cranial nerve nuclei does not support the different theories of head segmentation.

Acknowledgments. The works described in this endeavor was supported partly by the Hungarian National Research Fund and partly by research funds of the Ministry of Welfare.

References

Addens JL (1933) The motor nuclei and roots of the cranial and first spinal nerves of vertebrates. Z Anat Entw Gesch 101:307–410

Akert K, Glicksman MA, Lang W, Grob P, Huber A (1980) The Edinger-Westphal nucleus in the monkey. A retrograde tracer study. Brain Res 184:491–498

Ariëns Kappers CU, Huber GC, Crosby EC (1936) The comparative anatomy of the nervous system of vertebrates, including man. MacMillan, New York

Ashwell KW (1982) The adult mouse facial nerve nucleus: morphology and musculotopic organization. J Anat 135:531–538

Baisden RH, Woodruff ML, Whittington DL, Baker DC, Benson AE (1987) Cells of origin of the branches of the facial nerve: a retrograde HRP study in the rabbit. Am J Anat 178:175–184

Baker R, Highstein SM (1978) The vestibular projection to medial rectus subdivision of the oculomotor complex. J Neurphysiol 41:1629–1646

Baker RR, McCrea RA, Spencer FR (1980) Synaptic organization of cat accessory abducens nucleus. J Neurophysiol 43:771–791

Balfour FM (1878) A monograph on the development of elasmobranch fishes. MacMillan, London

Barbas-Henry HA (1982) The motor nuclei and primary projections of the facial nerve in the monitor lizard, *Varanus exanthematicus*. J Comp Neurol 207:105–113

Barbas-Henry HA, Lohman AHM (1984) The motor nuclei and primary projections of the IXth, Xth, XIth and XIIth cranial nerves in the monitor lizard, *Varanus exanthematicus*. J Comp Neurol 226:565–579

Barbas-Henry HA, Lohman AHM (1986) The motor complex and primary projections of the trigeminal nerve in the monitor lizard, *Varanus exanthematicus*. J Comp Neurol 254:314–329

Barbas-Henry HA, Lohman AHM (1988) The motor nuclei and sensory neurons of the IIIrd, IVth and VIth cranial nerves in the monitor lizard, *Varanus exanthematicus*. J Comp Neurol 267:370–386

Barry MA (1987) Central connections of the IXth and Xth cranial nerves in the clearnose skate, *Raja glanteria*. Brain Res 425:159–163

Batini C, Buisseret-Delmas C, Corvisier J (1976) Horseradish peroxidase localization of masticatory muscle motoneurons in cat. J Physiol (Paris) 72:301–309

Berkhoudt H, Klein BG, Zeigler HP (1982) Afferents to the trigeminal and facial motor nuclei in pigeon (*Columba livia L.*): central connections of jaw motoneurons. J Comp Neurol 209:301–312

Bieger D, Hopkins D (1987) Viscerotopic representation of the upper alimentary tract in the medulla oblongata in the rat: the nucleus ambiguus. J Comp Neurol 262:546–562

Blevin CE (1964) Studies on the innervation of the stapedius muscle of the cat. Anat Rec 149:157–172

Borg E (1973) On the neuronal organization of the acoustic middle ear reflex. A physiological and anatomical study. Brain Res 149:101–123

Burde RM, Loewy AD (1980) Central origins of oculomotor parasympathetic neurons in the monkey. Brain Res 198:434–439

Burde RM, Parelman JJ, Luskin M (1982) Lack of unity of Edinger-Westphal nucleus projections to the ciliary ganglion and spinal cord: a double labelling approach. Brain Res 249:379–382

Burde RM, Williams F (1989) Parasympathetic nuclei. Brain Res 498:371–375
Carlton SM, Chung JM, Leonard RB, Willis WD (1985) Funicular trajectories of brainstem neurons projecting to the lumbar spinal cord in the monkey (*Macaca fascicularis*): a retrograde labelling study. J Comp Neurol 241:382–404
Carpenter MB, Peter P (1970) Accessory oculomotor nuclei in the monkey. J Hirnforsch 12:405–418
Castiglioni AJ, Gallaway MC, Coulter JD (1978) Spinal projections from the midbrain in the monkey. J Comp Neurol 178:329–346
Chibuzo GA, Cummings F (1982) An enzyme trace study of the organization of the somatic motor center for the innervation of different muscles of the tongue: evidence for two sources. J Comp Neurol 205:273–281
Ciriello J, Calaresu FR (1982) Medullary origin of vagal preganglionic axons to the heart of the cat. J Auton Nerv Syst 5:9–22
Contreras RJ, Gomez MM, Norgren R (1980) Central origins of cranial nerve parasympathetic neurons in the rat. J Comp Neurol 190:373–394
Crompton AW (1989) The evolution of mammalian mastication. In: Wake DB, Roth G (eds) Complex organismal functions: integration and evolution in vertebrates. Wiley, Chichester, pp 23–40
Dom RM (1982) Topographical representation of the peripheral nerve branches of the facial nucleus of opossum. A study utilizing horseradish peroxidase. Brain Res 246: 281–284
Dubner R, Sessle BJ, Storey AT (1978) The neural basis of oral and facial function. Plenum, New York
DuBois F, Foley JO (1936) Experimental studies on the vagus and spinal accessory nerves in the cat. Anat Rec 64:285–307
Edinger L (1885) Über den Verlauf centralen Hirnnervenbahnen mit Demonstrationen von Präparaten. Arch Psychiatr Nervenkr 16:858–859
Erichsen JT, Reiner A, Karten HJ (1982) Co-occurrence of substance P-like and Leu-enkephalin-like immunoreactivities in neurons and fibers of avian nervous system. Nature 295:407–410
Evinger C, Graf WM, Baker R (1987) Extra- and intracellular HRP analysis of the organization of extraocular motoneurons and internuclear neurons in the guinea pig and rabbit. J Comp Neurol 252:429–444
Fahrenholz C (1937) Drüsen der Mundhöhle. In: Bolk L, Göppert E, Kallius E, Lubosch W (eds) Handbuch der vergleichenden Anatomie der Wirbeltiere, vol III. Darmsystem, Urban and Schwarzenberg, Berlin, pp 115–200
Flieger St (1964) Experimentelle Bestimmung der Lage und Ausdehnung des Kernes des N. Accessorius (XI) beim Schaf. Acta Anat 57:220–231
Flieger St (1966) Experimentelle Bestimmung der Lage und Ausdehnung des Kernes des N. Accessorius (XI) beim Pferd. Acta Anat 63:89–100
Flieger St (1967) Experimental determination of the topography and range of the nucleus nervi accessorii (XI) in the cow. J Hirnforsch 9:187–197
Friauf E, Baker R (1985) An intracellular HRP study of cat tensor tympani motoneurons. Exp Brain Res 57:499–511
Fritzsch B, Sonntag R, Dubuc R, Ohta Y, Grillner S (1990) Organization of the six motor nuclei innervating the ocular muscles in lamprey. J Comp Neurol 294:491–506
Froriep A (1902) Einige Bemerkungen zur Kopffrage. Anat Anz 21
Fürbringer M (1897) Über die spinooccipitalen Nerven der Selachier und Holocephalen und ihre vergleichende Morphologie. Festschr C Gegenbaur 3:349–788
Gacek RR (1975) Localization of laryngeal motor neurons in the kitten. Laryngoscope 85:1841–1861
Ganchrow D, Ganchrow JR, Gentle MJ (1986) Central afferent connections and origin of efferent projections of the facial nerve in the chicken (*Gallus gallus domesticus*). J Comp Neurol 248:455–463
Gannon PJ, Eden AR (1987) A specialized innervation of the tensor tympani muscle in Macaca fascicularis. Brain Res 404:257–262
Gans C, Northcutt RG (1983) Neural crest and the origin of vertebrates: a new head. Science 220:268–274

Gaupp E (1896) A. Ecker's und R. Wiedersheim's Anatomie des Frosches, vol I. Vieweg, Braunschweig, p 548
Gaupp E (1899) A. Ecker's und R. Wiedersheim's Anatomie des Frosches, vol II. Vieweg, Braunschweig, pp 144–146
Gaupp E (1904) A. Ecker's und R. Wiedersheim's Anatomie des Frosches, vol III. Vieweg, Braunschweig, pp 177–184
Gegenbaur O (1888) Die Matamerie des Kopfes und die Wirbeltheorie des Kopfskelettes. Gegenbaurs Morph Jahrb 13
Gestrin P, Sterling P (1977) Anatomy and physiology of the goldfish oculomotor system II. Firing patterns of neurons in the abducens nucleus and surrounding medulla and their relation to the eye movements. J Neurophysiol 40:573–588
Goethe JW (1824) Das Schödelgerüst aus sechs Wirbelknochen auferbaut; zur Naturwissenschaft überhaupt, besonders zur Morphologie, vol II. Stuttgart, Tübingen, pp 541–684
Gillaspy CC (1954) Experimental study of the cranial motor nuclei in reptilia. J Comp Neurol 100:481–510
Goodrich ES (1930) Studies on the structure and development of vertebrates. MacMillan, London
Görcs T, Antal M, Olah E, Székely G (1979) An improved cobalt labelling technique with complex compounds. Acta Biol Acad Sci Hung 30:79–86
Graf W, Brunker WJ (1984) Elasmobranch oculomotor organization: anatomical and theoretical aspects of the phylogenetic development of vestibulooculomotor connectivity. J Comp Neurol 227:569–581
Gray TS, McMaster SE, Hervey JA, Gormezano I (1981) Localization of retractor bulbi motoneurons in the rabbit. Brain Res 226:93–106
Green EC (1959) Anatomy of the rat. Hafner, New York
Guinan JJ Jr, Joseph MP, Norris BE (1989) Brainstem facial-motor pathways from two distinct groups of stapedius motoneurons in the cat. J Comp Neurol 287:134–144
Gwyn DG, Leslie RA, Hopkins DA (1985) Observations on the afferent and efferent organization of the vagus nerve and the innervation of the stomach in the squirrel monkey. J Comp Neurol 239:163–175
Haller von Hallerstein V (1934) Kranialnerven. In: Bolk L, Göppert E, Kallius E, Lubosch W (eds) Handbuch der Vergleichenden Anatomie der Wirbeltiere, vol II. Nervensystem. Urban and Schwarzenberg, Berlin, pp 541–684
Heaton MB, Wayne DB (1983) Patterns of extraocular innervation by the oculomotor complex in the chick. J Comp Neurol 216:245–252
Herring SW, Wineski LE, Anapol FC (1989) Neural organization of the masseter muscle in the pig. J Comp Neurol 280:563–576
Hinrichsen CFL, Watson CD (1984) The facial nucleus of the rat. Representation of facial muscles revealed by retrograde transport of horseradish peroxidase. Anat Rec 209:407–415
Holland PWH (1988) Homeobox genes and the vertebrate head. Development [Suppl] 103:17–24
Holomanova A, Cierny G, Zlatos J (1972) Localization of the motor cells of the spinal root of the accessory nerve in the cat. Folia Morphol (Praha) 20:232–234
Hopkins DA (1987) The dorsal motor nucleus of the vagus nerve and the nucleus ambiguus: structure and connections. In: Hainswarth R, McWillian PN, Mary DASG (eds) Cardiogenic reflexes. Oxford University Press, Oxford, pp 187–203
Hopkins DA, Armour JA (1982) Medullary cells of origin of physiologically indentified cardiac nerves in the dog. Brain Res Bull 8:359–365
Hopkins DA, Gootman PM, Gootman N, DiRusso SM, Zeballos ME (1984) Brainstem cell of origin of the cervical vagus and cardiopulmonary nerves in the neonatal pig (*Sus Scrofa*). Brain Res 360:63–72
Huber E (1930) Evolution of facial musculature and cutaneous fields of trigeminus. Quar Rev Biol 5:113–437
Hudson LC, Cummings JF (1985) The origins of innervation of the esophagus of the dog. Brain Res 326:125–136

Huxley Th (1858–59) On the theory of the vertebrate skull. Proc R Soc 9:381
Ibrahim Bin Haji Mohd Y, Leong SK (1979) Localization of neurons supplying the temporalis muscle in the rat and monkey. Neurosci Lett 11:63–68
Jacobson AG (1988) Somitomeres: mesodermal segments of vertebrate embryos. Development [Suppl] 104:209–220
Jacquin MF, Rhoades RW, Erfiejian HL, Egger MD (1983) Organization and morphology of masticatory neurons in the rat: a retrograde HRP study. J Comp Neurol 218:239–256
Joseph MP, Guinan JJ Jr, Fullerton BC, Norris BE, Kiang NYS (1985) Number and distribution of stapedius motoneurons in cat. J Comp Neurol 232:43–54
Kalia M, Mesulam MM (1980a) Brain stem projections of sensory and motor components of the vagus complex in the cat: I. The cervical vagus and nodose ganglion. J Comp Neurol 193:435–465
Kalia M, Mesulam MM (1980b) Brain stem projections of sensory and motor components of the vagus complex in the cat: II. Laryngeal, tracheobronchial, pulmonary, cardiac and gastrointestinal branches. J Comp Neurol 193:467–508
Kalia M, Sullivan JM (1982) Brainstem projections of sensory and motor components of the vagus nerve in the rat. J Comp Neurol 211:248–264
Katz DM, Karten HJ (1983) Subnuclear organization of the dorsal motor nucleus of the vagus nerve in the pigeon, *Columba livia*. J Comp Neurol 217:31–46
Keller JT, Saunders MC, Ongkiko CM, Johnson J, Frank E, van Loveren H, Tew JM Jr (1983) Identification of motoneurons innervating the tensor tympani and tensor veli palatini muscles in the cat. Brain Res 270:209–215
Kennedy MC (1981a) Motoneurons that control vocalization in a reptile: an HRP histochemical study. Brain Res 218:337–341
Kennedy MC (1981b) HRP localization of the hypoglossal nucleus in a lizard. Brain Res 218:331–336
Kimmel CB, Sepich DS, Trevarrow B (1988) Development of segmentation in zebrafish. Development [Suppl] 104:197–207
Kitamura S, Sakai A (1982) A study on the localization of the sternocleidomastoid and trapezius motoneurons in the rat by means of the HRP method. Anat Rec 202:527–636
Krammer EB, Lischka MF, Egger TP, Riedl M, Gruber H (1987) The motoneuronal organization of the spinal accessory nuclear complex. Adv Anat Embryol Cell Biol 103:1–62
Krammer EB, Rath T, Lischka MF (1979) Somatotopic organization of the hypoglossal nucleus: a HRP study in the rat. Brain Res 170:533–536
Kume M, Uemura M, Matsuda K, Matsushima R, Mizuno N (1978) Topographical representation of peripheral branches of the facial nerve within the facial nucleus a HRP study in the cat. Neurosci Lett 8:5–8
Labanderia-Gracia JL, Segade LAG, Saurez-Nunez JM (1983) Localization of motoneurons supplying the extraocular muscles of the rat using horseradish peroxidase and fluorescent double labelling. J Anat 137:247–262
Labanderia-Gracia JL, Guerra-Seijis MJ, Segade LAG, Suarez-Nunez JM (1983) Identification of abducens motoneurons, accessory abducens motoneurons, and abducens internuclear neurons in the chick by retrograde transport of horseradish peroxidase. J Comp Neurol 259:140–149
Landgren S, Olsson KA (1976) Localization of evoked potentials in the digastric, masseteric, supra- and infratrigeminal subnuclei of the cat. Exp Brain Res 26:299–318
Lawn AM (1966a) The localization in the nucleus ambiguus of the rabbit, of the cells of origin of motor nerve fibers in the glossopharyngeal nerve and various branches of the vagus nerve by means of retrograde degeneration. J Comp Neurol 127:293–306
Lawn AM (1966b) The nucleus ambiguus of the rabbit. J Comp Neurol 127:307–320
Le Douarin N (1982) The neural crest. University Press, London
Limwongse V, DeSantis M (1977) Cell body locations and axonal pathway of neurons innervating muscles of mastication in the rat. Am J Anat 149:477–488
Linden RWA (1978) Properties of intraoral mechanoreceptors represented in the mesencephalic nucleus of the fifth nerve in the cat. J Physiol (Lond.) 279:395–408

Loewy AD, Saper CB (1978) Edinger-Westphal nucleus: projections to the brain stem and spinal cord in the cat. Brain Res 150:1–27

Lubosch W (1938) Muskeln des Kopfes. Viscerale Muskulatur. In: Bolk L, Göppert E, Kallius E, Lubosch W (eds) Handbuch der vergleichenden Anatomie der Wirbeltiere, vol V, Skelettsystem, Muskelsystem, Urogenitalsystem. Urban and Schwarzenberg, Berlin, pp 1011–1104

Luiten PGM, Dijkstra-de Vlieger HP (1978) Extraocular muscle representation of the carp. J Comp Neurol 179:669–676

Lund JP, Olsson KA (1983) The importance of reflexes and their control during jaw movement. TINS 6:458–463

Lupin AJ (1969) The relationship of tensor palati and tensor tympani muscles. Arch Otolaryngol 78:792–796

Luschei ES, Goldberg LS (1981) Neural mechanisms of mandibular control: mastication and biting. In: Brooks NB (ed) Handbook of Physiology, vol II (Nervous System). American Physiological Society, Bethesda, Maryland, pp 1237–1274

Lyon MJ (1978) The central locations of the motor neurons to the stapedius muscle in cat. Brain Res 143:437–444

Maciewicz R, Phipps BS, Foote WE, Eronin N, Difiglia M (1983) Distribution of substance P-containing neurons in the cat Edinger-Westphal nucleus: relationship to efferent projection systems. Brain Res 270:217–230

Maciewicz R, Phipps BS, Grenier J, Poletti CE (1984) Edinger-Westphal nucleus cholecystokinin immunocytochemistry and projections to spinal cord and trigeminal nucleus in the cat. Brain Res 299:139–145

Marinesco G, Parhon C (1917) Recherches sur les noyaux moteurs d'origine du nerf pneumogastrique et sur les localisations dans ces noyaux. J Neurologie 12: 61–77

Matesz C (1983) Termination areas of primary afferent fibers of the trigeminal nerve in the rat. Acta Biol Hung 34:31–44

Matesz C (1983) The structure of the motor and sensory cranial nerve nuclei in the frog and rat. (In Hungarian) Thesis, University of Debrecen

Matesz C (1990a) Development of the abducens nuclei in *Xenopus laevis*. Dev Brain Res 51:179–184

Matesz C (1990b) Development of the oculomotor and trochlear nuclei in the *Xenopus* toad. Neurosci Lett 116:1–6

Matesz C, Hevessy Zs (to be published) Localization and morphology of motoneurons innervating the jaw muscles of a frog, *Rana esculenta*. Neurosci Lett

Matesz C, Székely G (1977) The dorsomedial nuclear group of cranial nerves in the frog. Acta Biol Acad Sci Hung 28:461–474

Matesz C, Székely G (1978) The motor column and sensory projections of the branchial cranial nerves in the frog. J Comp Neurol 178:157–176

Matesz C, Székely G (1983) The motor nuclei of the glossopharyngeal-vagal and the accessory nerves in the rat. Acta Biol Hung 34:215–230

Matsuda K, Uemura M, Takeuchi Y, Kume M, Matsushima R, Mizuno N (1979) Localization of motoneurons innervating the posterior belly of digastric muscle: a comparative anatomical study by the HRP method Neurosci Lett 12:47–52

Meesson H, Olszewski J (1949) A cytoarchitectonic atlas of the rhombencephalon of the rabbit. Karger, Basel

Meier SP (1979) Development of the chick mesoblast. Formation of the embryonic axis establishment of the metameric pattern. Dev Biol 73:25–45

Meier SP (1982) The development of segmentation in the cranial region of vertebrate embryos. Scanning Electron Microsc 3:1269–1282

Miyazaki T, Yoshida Y, Hirano T, Kanaseki S (1981) Central location of the motoneurons supplying the thyrohyoid and the geniohyoid muscles as demonstrated by horseradish peroxidase method. Brain Res 219:423–427

Mizuno N, Konishi A, Sato M (1975) Localization of masticatory motoneurons in the cat and rat by means of retrograde axonal transport of horseradish peroxidase. J Comp Neurol 164:105–116

Mizuno N, Matsuda K, Iwahori N, Uemura-Sumi M, Kume M, Matsushima R (1981) Representation of the masticatory muscles in the motor trigeminal nucleus of the macaque monkey. Neurosci Lett 21:19–22

Mizuno N, Nomura S, Konishi A, Uemura-Sumi M, Takahashi O, Yasui Y, Takada M, Matsushima R (1982) Localization of motoneurons innervating the tensor tympani muscles and horseradish peroxidase study in the guinea pig and cat. Neurosci Lett 31:205–208

Molhant M (1912) Le nerf vague. Etude anatomique et experimental. Deuxième partie. Le noyau ambigu, les connexions anatomique et la valeur fonctionnelle du noyau central du vague et du noyau ambigu. Nevraxe 13:9–316

Moody SA, Meszler RM (1980) Subnuclear organization of the ophidian trigeminal motor nucleus. I. Localization of neurons and synaptic bouton distribution. J Comp Neurol 190:463–486

Morita Y, Finger ThE (1987) Topographic representation of the sensory and motor roots of the vagus nerve in the medulla of goldfish, *Carassius auratus*. J Comp Neurol 264:231–249

Murphy EH, Garone M, Tashayyod D, Baker RR (1986) Innervation of extraocular muscles in the rabbit. J Comp Neurol 254:78–90

Narayanan CH, Narayanan Y (1976) An experimental inquiry into the central source of preganglionic fibers to the chick ciliary ganglion. J Comp Neurol 166:101–110

Naujoks-Manteuffel C, Manteuffeel G, Himstedt W (1986) Localization of motoneurons innervating the extraocular muscles in *Salamandra salamandra L.* (Amphibia, Urodela). J Comp Neurol 254:133–141

Nishi M (1938) B Augenmuskulatur. In: Bolk L, Göppert E, Kallius E, Lubosch W (eds) Handbuch der vergleichenden Anatomie der Wirbeltiere, vol V. Skelettsystem, Muskelsystem, Urogenitalsystem. Urban and Schwarzenberg, Berlin, pp 453–466

Noden DM (1983) The embryonic origins of avian cephalic and cervical muscles and associated connective tissues. Am J Anat 168:257–276

Nomura S, Mizuno N (1983) Axonal trajectories of masticatory motoneurons genu formation of axons of jaw-opening motoneurons in the cat. Neurosci Lett 37:11–15

Nosaka S, Yamamoto T, Yasunaga K (1979) Localization of vagus cardioinhibitory preganglionic neurons within rat brain stem. J Comp Neurol 186:79–92

Oka Y, Takeuchi H, Satou M, Ueda K (1987a) Cobaltic lysine study of the morphology and distribution of the cranial nerve efferent neurons (motoneurons and preganglionic parasympathetic neurons) and rostral spinal motoneurons in the Japanese toad. J Comp Neurol 259:400–423

Oka Y, Takeuchi H, Satou M, Ueda K (1987b) Morphology and distribution of the preganglionic parasympathetic neurons of the facial, glossopharyngeal and vagus nerves in the Japanese toad: a cobaltic lysine study. Brain Res 400:389–395

Oken L (1807) Über die Bedeutung der Schädelknochen. Jena

Okubo J, Kitamura S, Ogata K, Sokai A (1987) Localization of rabbit laryngeal motoneurons in the nucleus ambiguus. Exp Neurol 96:528–539

Olszewski J, Baxter D (1954) Cytoarchitecture of the human brain stem. Karger, Basel

Parver LM, Auker ChR, Carpenter DO, Doyle Th (1982) Choroidal blood flow. II. Reflexive control in the monkey. Arch Ophthalmol (Chicago) 100:1327–1330

Pilar G, Tuttle JB (1982) Model cholinergic synapses. In: Hanin J, Goldberg AM (eds) Progress in modern cholinergic biology. Raven, New York, pp 213–247

Porter JD, Guthrei BL, Sparks DL (1983) Innervation of monkey extraocular muscles. Localization of sensory and motor neurons by retrograde transport of horseradish peroxidase. J Comp Neurol 218:208–219

Prechtl JC, Powley TL (1985) Organization and distribution of the rat subdiaphragmatic vagus and associated paraganglia. J Comp Neurol 235:182–195

Ramón Y, Cajal S (1909) Histologie du système nerveux de homme et des vertèbres, vol 1. Maloine, Paris

Rapoport S (1978) Location of sternocleidomastoid and trapezius motoneurons in the cat. Brain Res 156:339–344

Reiner A, Karten HJ, Gamlin PDR, Erichsen JT (1983) Parasympathetic ocular control. Functional subdivisions and circuitry of the avian nucleus of Edinger-Westphal. TINS 6:140–145

Romanes GJ (194) The spinal accessory nerve in the sheep. J Anat 74:336–347

Roth G, Nishikawa K, Dicke U, Wake DB (1988) Topography and cytoarchitecture of the motor nuclei in the brainstem of salamanders. J Comp Neurol 278:181–194

Roth G, Wake DB (1985) The structure of the brainstem and cervical spinal cord in lungless salamanders (family Plethodontidae) and its relation to feeding. J Comp Neurol 241:99–110

Roth G, Wake DB, Wake MH, Rettig G (1984) Distribution of accessory and hypoglossal nerves in the hindbrain and spinal cord of lungless salamanders, family Plethodontidae. Neurosci Lett 44:53–57

Ruskell GL (1971) Facial parasympathetic innervation of the choroidal blood vessels in monkeys. Exp Eye Res 12:166–172

Sakai Y (1987) Neurulation in the mouse. I. The ontogenesis of neural segments and the determination of topographical regions in a central nervous system. Anat Rec 218:450–457

Satomi H, Takahashi K, Aoki M, Kasaba T, Kurosawa Y, Otsuka K (1985) Localization of the spinal accessory motoneurons in the cervical cord in connection with the phrenic nucleus: an HRP study in cats. Brain Res 344:227–230

Schnyder H (1984) The innervation of the monkey accessory lateral rectus muscle. Brain Res 296:139–244

Schwab MA (1979) Variation in the rhombencephalon. In: Gans C, Northcutt RG, Ulinski PS (eds) Biology of the reptilia, vol 10. Academic, San Francisco, pp 201–246

Schwitzer H, Ruebsamen R, Ruehle C (1981) Localization of brain stem motoneurons innervating the laryngeal muscles in the rufous horseshoe bat, *Rhinolophus Rouxi*. Brain Res 230:41–50

Shaw MD, Baker R (1983) The localizations of stapedius and tensor tympani motoneurons in the cat. J Comp Neurol 216:10–19

Shaw MD, Baker R (1985) Morphology of motoneurons in a mixed motor pool of the cat facial nucleus that innervate orbicularis oculi and quadratus labii superioris, stained intracellularly with horseradish peroxidase. Neuroscience 14:627–643

Soliman MA (1964) Die Kopfnerven der Schildkröten. Z Wiss Zool 169:216–312

Spangler KM, Henkel CK, Miller IJ Jr (1982) Location of the motor neurons to the tensor tympani muscle. Neurosci Lett 32:23–27

Spencer RF, Baker RR, McCrea RA (1980) Localization and morphology of cat retractor bulbi motoneurons. J Neurophysiol 43:754–770

Spencer RF, Porter JD (1981) Innervation and structure of extraocular muscles in the monkey in comparison to those of the cat. J Comp Neurol 198:649–665

Starck D (1978) Vergleichende Anatomie der Wirbeltiere auf evolutionsbiologische Grundlage. Theoretische Grundlagen, Stammesgeschichte und Systematik, vol I. Springer, Berlin Heidelberg New York

Starck D (1979) Vergleichende Anatomie der Wirbeltiere auf evolutionsbiologische Grundlage. Das Skeletensystem. Skelett der Wirbeltiere einschliesslich Lokomotionstypen, vol II. Springer, Berlin Heidelberg New York

Starck D (1982) Vergleichende Anatomie der Wirbeltiere, auf evolutionsbiologische Grundlage. Organe des aktiven Bewegungsapparates, der Koordination, der Umweltbeziehung, des Stoffwechsels und der Fortpflanzung, vol III. Springer, Berlin Heidelberg New York

Sterling P (1977) Anatomy and physiology of goldfish oculomotor system. I. Structure of abducens nucleus. J Neurophysiol 40:557–572

Strassman A, Mason P, Eckerstein F, Baughman RW, Maciewitz R (1987) Choline acetyltransferase immunocytochemistry of Edinger-Westphal and ciliary ganglion afferent neurons in the cat. Brain Res 423:293–304

Stuesse SL (1982) Origins of cardiac vagal preganglionic fibers: A retrograde transport study. Brain Res 236:15–25

Stuesse LS, Cruce LRC, Powell KS (1984) Organization within the cranial IX–X complex in ranid frogs: a horseradish peroxidase transport study. J Comp Neurol 222:358–365

Stuesse LS, Cruce LRC, Powell KS (1983) Afferent and efferent components of the hypoglossal nerve in the grass frog (*Rana pipiens*). J Comp Neurol 217:432–439

Sugimoto T, Itoh K, Mizuno N (1978) Direct projections from the Edinger-Westphal nucleus to the cerebellum and spinal cord in the cat: an HRP study. Neurosci Lett 9:17–22

Szabo T, Blasher S, Denizot J-P, Ravaille-Véron M (1991) The olfactoretinalis system-terminal nerve? Neuroreport 2:73–76

Szabo T, Lázár G, Libouban S, Tóth P, Ravaille M (1987) Oculomotor system of the waekly electric fish, *Gnathonemus petersii*. J Comp Neurol 264:480–493

Székely G (1976) The morphology of motoneurons and dorsal root fibers in the frog's spinal cord. Brain Res 103:275–290

Székely G,. Gallyas F (1975) Intensification of cobaltous sulphide precipitate in frog nervous tissue. Acta Biol Acad Sci Hung 26:175–188

Székely G, Matesz C (1982) The accessory motor nuclei of the trigeminal, facial and abducens nerves in the rat. J Comp Neurol 210:258–264

Székely G, Matesz C (1987) Trigeminal motoneurons with disparate dendritic geometry innervate different muscle groups in the frog. Neurosci Lett 77:161–165

Székely G, Matesz C (1988) Topography and organization of cranial nerve nuclei in the sand lizard, *Lacerta agilis*. J Comp Neurol 267:525–544

Szentágothai J (1942) Die zentrale Leitungsbahn des Lichtreflexes der Pupillen. Arch Psychiatr 115:136–156

Szentágothai J (1943) Die Lokalisation der Kehlkopfmuskulatur in den Vaguskernen. Z Anat Entw Gesch 112:704–710

Szentágothai J (1949) Functional representation of the motor trigeminal nucleus. J Comp Neurol 90:111–120

Taber E (1961) The cytoarchitecture of the brainstem of the cat. I. Brainstem nuclei of the cat. J Comp Neurol 116:27–69

Takahashi O, Mizuno N, Mitani A, Takeuchi Y, Matsushima R (1984) Identification of motoneurons innervating the tensor tympani muscle in the rabbit: a retrograde horseradish peroxidase study. Neurosci Lett 49:19–23

Thompson GC, Igarashi M, Stach BA (1985) Identification of stapedius muscle motoneurons in squirrel monkey and bush baby. J Comp Neurol 231:270–279

Tomanes GJ (1940) The spinal accessory nerve in the ship. J Anat 74:336–347

Toyoshima K, Kawana E, Sakai H (1980) On the neuronal origin of the afferents to the ciliary ganglion in cat. Brain Res 185:67–76

Uemura-Sumi M, Mizuno N, Nomura S, Iwahori N, Takeuchi Y, Matsushima R (1981) Topographical representation of the hypoglossal nerve branches and tongue muscles in the hypoglossal nucleus of macaque monkeys. Neurosci Lett 22:31–35

Urban L, Székely G (1983) Intracellular staining of motoneurons with complex cobalt compounds in the frog. J Neurobiol 14:157–161

Vacher SR, Guinan JJ Jr, Koble JB (1989) Intracellularly labelled stapedus-motoneuron cell bodies in the cat are spatially organized according to their physiologic responses. J Comp Neurol 289:401–415

van Gehuchten A (1898a) Recherches sur l'origine réelle des nerfs craniens. I. Les nerfs moteurs oculaires. J Neurol 3:114–129

van Gehuchten A. (1898b) Recherches sur l'origine réelle des nerfs craniens. II. Nerf facial (suite) J Neurol 3:293–303

van Loveren H, Saunder MC, Keller JT (1983) Localization of motoneurons innervating the levator veli palatini muscle in the cat. Brain Res Bull 11:303–307

van Loveren H, Saunders MC, Cassini P, Keller JT (1985) Localization of motoneurons innervating the stylopharyngeus muscle in the cat. Neurosci Lett 58:251–255

Wake BD, Nishikawa C, Dicke U, Roth G (1988) Organization of the motor nuclei in the cervical spinal cord of salamanders. J Comp Neurol 278:195–208

Warwick R (1954) The ocular parasympathetic nerve supply and its mesencephalic sources. J Anat (Lond.) 88:71–93

Wathey JC (1988) Identification of the teleost Edinger-Westphal nucleus by horseradish peroxidase labelling and by electrophysiological criteria. J Comp Physiol (A) 162:511–514

Welt C, Abbs JH (1990) Musculotopic organization of the facial motor nucleus in *Macaca fascicularis*: a morphometric and retrograde tracing study with cholera toxin B-HRP. J Comp Neurol 291:621–636

Westphal C (1887) Uber einen Fall von chronischer progressiver Lähmung der Augenmuskeln (Ophthalmoplegia externa) nebst Beschreibung von Ganglienzellengruppen im Bereiche des Oculomotoriuskerns. Arch Psychiatr Nervenheilk 98:846–871

Wild JM, Zeigler HP (1980) Central representation and somatotopic organization of the jaw muscles within the facial and trigeminal nuclei of the pigeon (*Columba livia*). J Comp Neurol 192:175–201

Willard WA (1915) The cranial nerves of *Anolis carolinensis*. Bull Mus Comp Zool Harv 59:15–11

Yoshida Y, Miyazaki T, Hirano M, Shin T, Totoki T, Kanaseki T (1981) Localization of efferent neurons innervating the pharyngeal constrictor muscles and the cervical esophagus muscle in the cat by means of the horseradish peroxidase method. Neurosci Lett 22:91–95

Yoshida Y, Tsuru K, Mitsuhiro Y, Otani K, Shigenaga Y (1987) Morphology of masticatory motoneurons stained intracellularly with horseradish peroxidase. Brain Res 316:393–401

Youn BW, Malacinski GM (1981) Comparative analysis of amphibian somite morphogenesis: cell rearrangement patterns during rosette formation and myoblast fusion. J Embryol Exp Morph 66:1–26

Subject Index